Color Atlas of

HEART FAILURE

Second Edition

Leonard M Shapiro BSc, MD, FRCP, FACC

Consultant Cardiologist
Papworth and Addenbrooke's Hospital
Cambridge, UK

ℳ Mosby-Wolfe

Copyright © 1995 Times Mirror International Publishers Limited

Published in 1995 by Mosby-Wolfe, an imprint of Times Mirror International Publishers Limited

Printed by Grafos S.A. Arte Sobel papel, Barcelona, Spain

ISBN 0 7234 1899 3

For full details of all Times Mirror International Publishers Limited titles, please write to Times Mirror International Publishers Limited, Lynton House, 7–12 Tavistock Square, London WC1H 9LB, England.

A CIP catalogue record for this book is available from the British Library.

CONTENTS

Acknowledgements iv

Preface v

1 Heart Failure 7
Definition of heart failure 7
Epidemiology of heart failure 8
Clinical manifestations of heart failure 11
Investigations in heart failure 16
Causes of deterioration of heart failure 19
Causes of heart failure 24

2 Coronary Artery Disease 25
Poor left ventricular function 25
Mitral regurgitation 35
Ventricular septal defect 39
Left ventricular aneurysm 41
Right ventricular infarction 46

3 Valvular Heart Disease 49
Chronic mitral valve disease 49
Chronic aortic valve disease 65
Tricuspid valve disease 82
Heart failure following cardiac surgery 87

4 Heart Muscle Disease 93
Idiopathic dilated cardiomyopathy 94
Hypertrophic cardiomyopathy 101
Restrictive cardiomyopathy and
endomyocardial fibrosis 111
Other causes of heart muscle disease 117

5 Hypertension 123

6 Pericardial Disease 129
Constriction 129
Cardiac tamponade 132

7 Infection and Heart Failure 137
Infective endocarditis 137

8 Cardiac Tumours 143

9 Congenital Heart Disease 145
Atrial septal defect 145
Ventricular septal defect 148
Coarctation of the aorta 150

10 Pulmonary Hypertension 153
Pulmonary embolism 155

References 157

Index 158

ACKNOWLEDGEMENTS

I am indebted to the many colleagues and friends who contributed the illustrations for the first and second editions. I wish to thank Dr Kim Fox the co-author of the first edition and Mrs Pat Mainwood who typed the manuscript.

PREFACE

Breathlessness is a common cardiac symptom. This atlas of heart failure contains colour photographs of the pathology and investigation of patients suffering from both the common and uncommon causes of this condition. This book is divided into 10 sections and every attempt has been made to be as comprehensive as possible. This atlas is primarily aimed at undergraduates, postgraduates studying for higher diplomas, physicians and general practitioners, who manage patients with heart disease.

This second edition has been extensively revised to include the new developments in the study and management of heart failure.

1. HEART FAILURE

Definition of heart failure

Heart failure is the pathophysiological state in which abnormal cardiac function leads to the delivery of blood at an inadequate rate for the requirements of the tissues. Such impairment of pump function often occurs with abnormally depressed myocardial contraction and it is frequently associated with an elevated filling pressure. The clinical syndrome of heart failure may occur with apparently normal myocardial function: in these circumstances a normal heart may fail if presented with a load that exceeds its capacity or when ventricular filling is impaired.

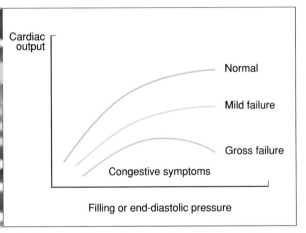

1 In the normal heart there remains a constant relationship between ventricular output (cardiac output) and filling pressure (end-diastolic pressure). In a failing heart the cardiac output fails to rise with increased filling pressure leading to congestive symptoms.

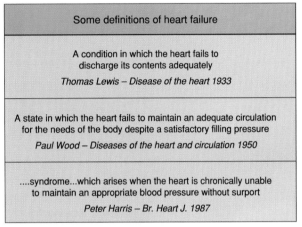

2 Heart failure may be defined in a number of ways.

Some definitions of heart failure
A condition in which the heart fails to discharge its contents adequately *Thomas Lewis – Disease of the heart 1933*
A state in which the heart fails to maintain an adequate circulation for the needs of the body despite a satisfactory filling pressure *Paul Wood – Diseases of the heart and circulation 1950*
....syndrome...which arises when the heart is chronically unable to maintain an appropriate blood pressure without surport *Peter Harris – Br. Heart J. 1987*

Criteria of CHF
Major criteria
Paroxysmal nocturnal dyspnoea or orthopnoea Neck-vein distention Rales Cardiomegaly Acute pulmonary oedema S3 gallop Increased venous pressure – > 16 cm of water Circulation time 25 sec. Hepatojugular reflux
Minor criteria
Ankle oedema Night cough Dyspnoea on exertion Hepatomegaly Pleural effusion Vital capacity ↓ 1/3 from maximum Tachycardia (rate of 120/min)
Major or minor criterion
Weight loss > 4.5 kg in 5 days in response to treatment

3 For epidemiological purposes, the Framingham heart study defined congestive heart failure as two major or one major plus two minor criteria (McKee *et al.*, 1971).

Epidemiology of heart failure

During the twentieth century, heart failure has remained one of the primary unresolved problems of cardiology and is a principal complication of virtually all forms of cardiac pathology. The incidence of most cardiovascular disorders has declined in western countries in the past 10–20 years. In contrast, the prevalence and incidence of congestive heart failure has increased.

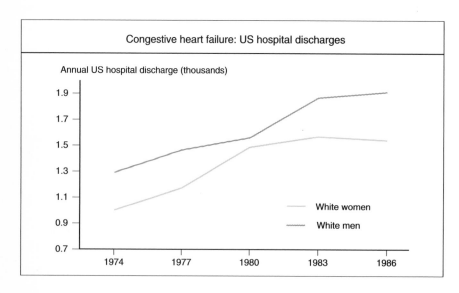

4 Heart failure is the most common hospital discharge diagnosis for patients over the age of 65 years and the number of admissions for this condition has risen threefold during the last 15 years. The number of cases of congestive heart failure will probably continue to rise as patients who previously would have died from acute myocardial infarction now survive with impaired left ventricular function (Ghali *et al.*, 1990).

5

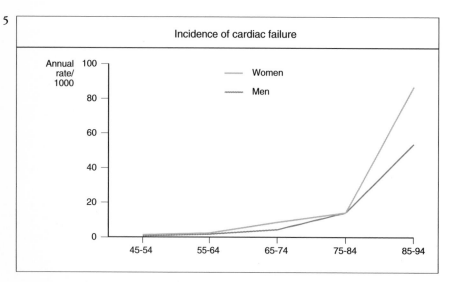

5 & 6 The Framingham study examined the incidence and natural history of heart failure in a cohort of 5200 persons over a 30-year period. Overt congestive heart failure (diagnosed on clinical and radiological signs) developed in 461 persons. The commonest causes were hypertension, and coronary and rheumatic heart disease. The incidence of heart failure rises steeply with age (**5**, Kannel *et al.*, 1988). The poor prognosis associated with the diagnosis of congestive heart failure is shown compared to matched controls (**6**, Kannel *et al.*, 1988).

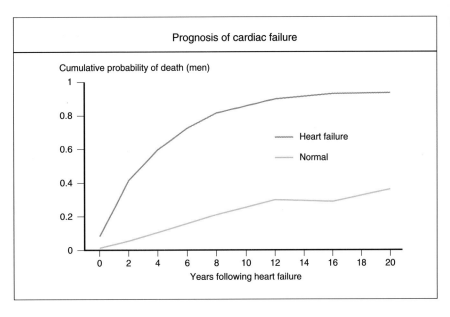

Prognosis of cardiac failure

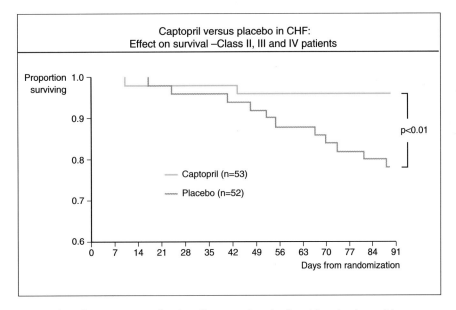

Captopril versus placebo in CHF:
Effect on survival –Class II, III and IV patients

7 A number of more recent studies (usually comparing placebo with active therapy) have examined the medium- and long-term mortality associated with the diagnosis of heart failure. Almost 20 per cent of patients with congestive heart failure die within three months (Newman *et al.*, 1988).

8

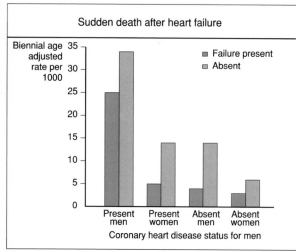

Sudden death after heart failure

Biennial age adjusted rate per 1000

■ Failure present
■ Absent

Coronary heart disease status for men

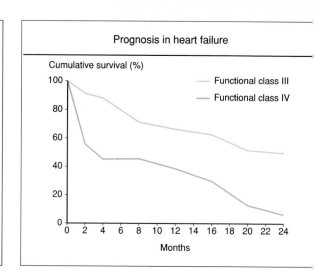

Prognosis in heart failure

Cumulative survival (%)

— Functional class III
— Functional class IV

Months

10

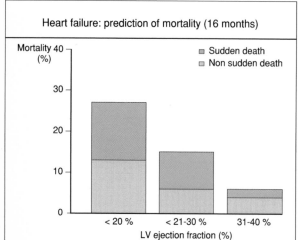

Heart failure: prediction of mortality (16 months)

Mortality (%)

■ Sudden death
■ Non sudden death

LV ejection fraction (%)

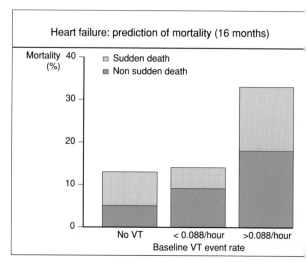

Heart failure: prediction of mortality (16 months)

Mortality (%)

■ Sudden death
■ Non sudden death

Baseline VT event rate

8–11 Death in patients with heart failure may result from deterioration in the underlying cardiac disease but more commonly death is sudden and presumably due to arrhythmias. Various factors determine the prognosis in heart failure including the underlying cardiac pathology, the presenting functional class and ventricular arrhythmias. The Framingham study shows the risk of sudden death in men and women with a history of heart failure or with failure present is considerably increased in the presence of coronary disease (**8**, Kannel *et al.,* 1988). Mortality is significantly related to functional class at presentation. Patients in NYHA class IV (dyspnoea at rest) have a worse two-year survival than those in NYHA III (**9**, Wilson, 1983). The resting left ventricular ejection fraction at presentation predicts short-term prognosis: patients with an ejection fraction of less than 20 per cent demonstrated a significantly greater mortality for both sudden death and non-sudden death compared to those with less impaired left ventricular function (**10**, Gradman, 1989). The presence of ventricular extrasystoles and tachycardia may be useful in predicting mortality in heart failure. Ambulatory electrocardiogram (ECG) recordings demonstrate that those with more baseline ventricular arrhythmias have the greatest mortality (**11**, Gradman, 1989).

Clinical manifestations of heart failure

Heart failure may manifest itself in a number of ways as a result of inadequate forward output or obstructed ventricular inflow. The former leads to 'forward failure' and the latter to 'backward failure'. The concept of 'backward failure' was first proposed in 1832 by James Hope who related these congestive symptoms to the increase in atrial and venous pressure when the ventricle was unable to discharge its contents. In 1913, MacKenzie proposed the 'forward failure' concept in which impaired arterial blood delivery related to the clinical manifestations. While initially there were opposing views concerning the pathogenesis of the different directions of heart failure, and in certain cases pure forms may be observed, both mechanisms operate in most patients with heart failure.

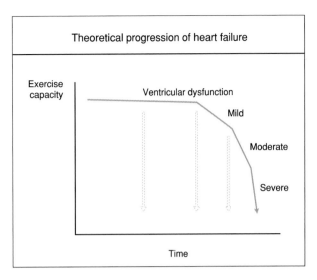

12 The theoretical natural history of heart failure, from asymptomatic ventricular dysfunction through progressive impairment of exercise capacity to the clinical syndrome of heart failure.

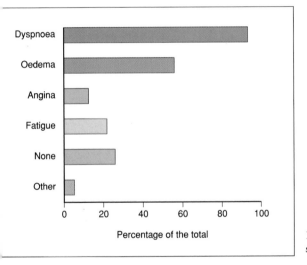

13 While some patients with congestive heart failure have no symptoms, the predominant presenting feature is breathlessness.

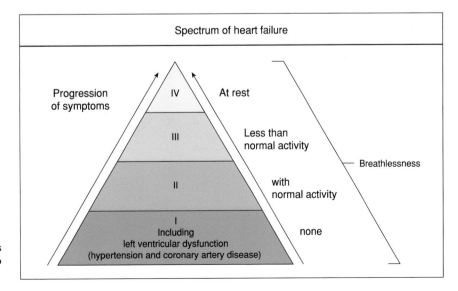

14 Breathlessness may present as mild exertional (class 1), through to dyspnoea at rest (class IV).

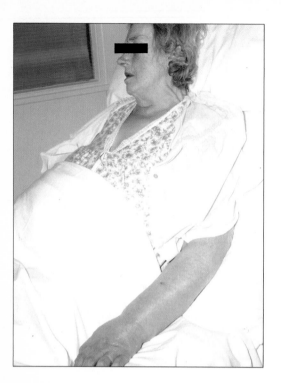

15 With worsening dyspnoea, orthopnoea and paroxysmal nocturnal dyspnoea may ensue, as in this case of an oedematous woman in heart failure sitting upright in bed.

16

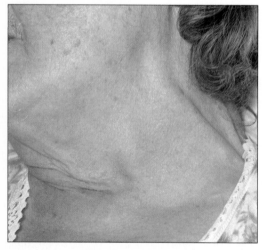

17

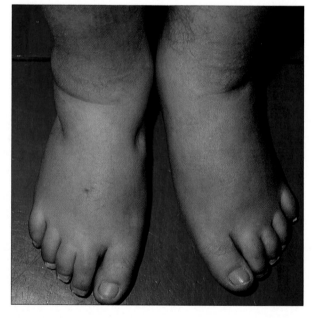

16 & 17 An elevated jugular venous pressure reflects raised right atrial pressure which in turn may be due to an elevated right ventricular filling pressure and right ventricular failure (**16**). Peripheral oedema is a cardinal feature of congestive heart failure, though it may occur in other conditions. Typically, oedema will pit on pressure (**17**).

18 Fatigue and weakness are non-specific but frequently reported symptoms in patients with a reduced cardiac output. Congestive heart failure may be associated with a reduction in bulk and histological and biochemical changes in skeletal muscle. The presence of oedema may mask the gross loss of muscle mass due to cardiac cachexia.

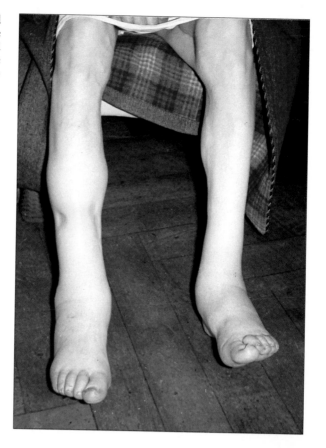

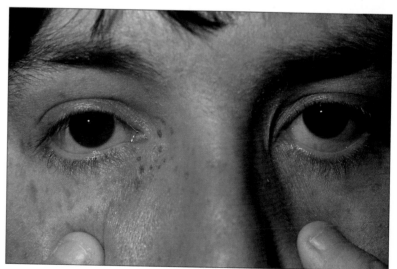

19 Other manifestations of severe heart failure include hepatic congestion and jaundice, as seen here, as well as hydrothorax, ascites and gastrointestinal symptoms.

20

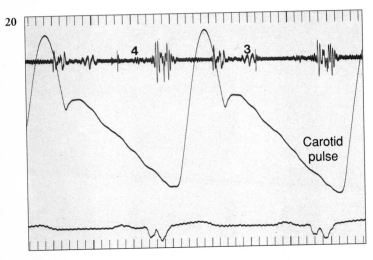

Carotid
pulse

21

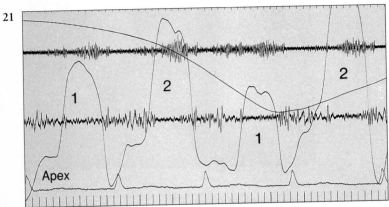

Apex

22

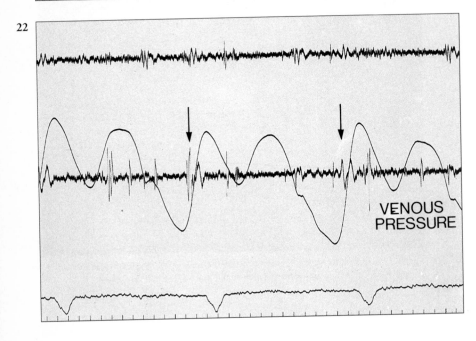

VENOUS
PRESSURE

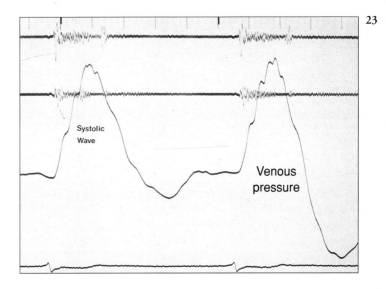

23

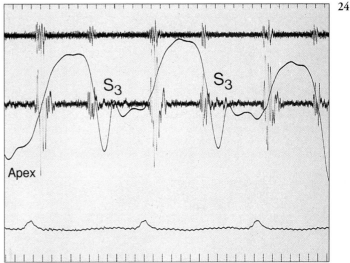

24

20–24 The physical findings vary with the severity of heart failure, its cause, and the relative involvement of right and left ventricles. A series of indirect pressure recordings and phonocardiograms are shown to illustrate the physical signs. The pulse in heart failure is typically of small volume and ill-sustained (**20**). When the patient develops increasing left ventricular failure, pulsus alternans may be present: alternate small (1) and large (2) beats which may be best elicited by the sphygmomanometer. In this example (**21**), the underlying cause of heart failure was aortic valve disease. The jugular venous pressure becomes elevated (**22**). The dominance of wave or descent varies with aetiology but with the onset of tricuspid regurgitation, the systolic wave is prominent (**23**). Cardiomegaly may be detected clinically. Following the development of widespread damage, left ventricular cavity dilatation will occur with outward and downward displacement of the apex, which cannot be distinguished from other causes of left ventricular dilatation. Auscultation at the apex reveals a third sound which may be palpable (**24**). A third and fourth heart sound may be demonstrated (**20**) and when there is a tachycardia, summation of the third and fourth heart sound (arrows) results in a typical gallop rhythm (**22**).

Investigations in heart failure

Investigations in heart failure should be directed towards the detection of a reversible aetiology or cause of deterioration. Investigation will also reveal the severity of the disease.

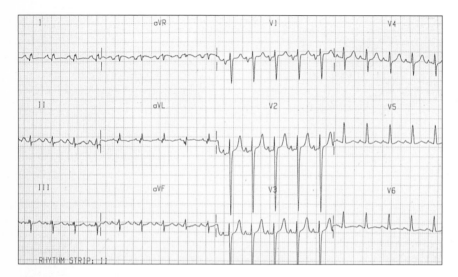

25 The electrocardiogram is often non-specific but may reflect the underlying aetiology such as hypertension or coronary heart disease. Gross left ventricular hypertrophy (deep S waves in V_{1-2} and tall R waves in V_{5-6} with lateral ST depression and T inversion ('strain pattern')) in atrial fibrillation is shown in a patient with heart failure due to hypertension.

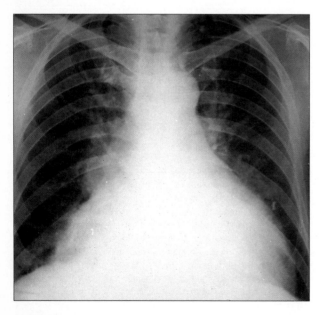

26 The chest radiograph is also non-specific but will usually reveal cardiomegaly with pulmonary vascular congestion or oedema, as in this example.

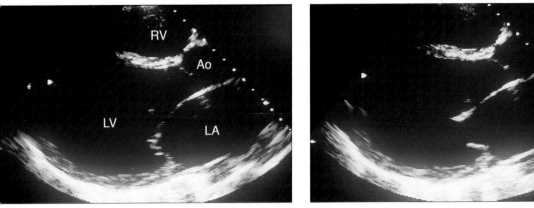
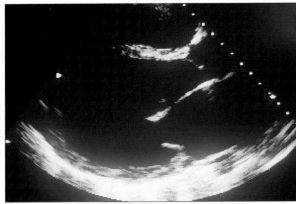

27 & 28 The echocardiogram has revolutionized the investigation of heart failure. The most frequently encountered findings are a dilated poorly contracting left ventricle with secondary atrial and right ventricular enlargement. This is the end-stage of a variety of disease processes. A long axis parasternal view (systole, **27**; diastole, **28**) of a dilated and poorly contracting left ventricle is shown. Much less commonly, a small hypertrophied left ventricle may be seen (as in hypertrophic cardiomyopathy, hypertension or amyloid heart disease) in which abnormal diastolic properties lead to the clinical manifestations of heart failure. The echocardiogram may show the aetiological basis of heart failure such as a left ventricular aneurysm or ventricular septal defect, valve disease or tumour, or complications such as pericardial effusion or mural thrombus (see later chapters). RV= right ventricle; Ao = aorta; LV = left ventricle; LA = left atrium.

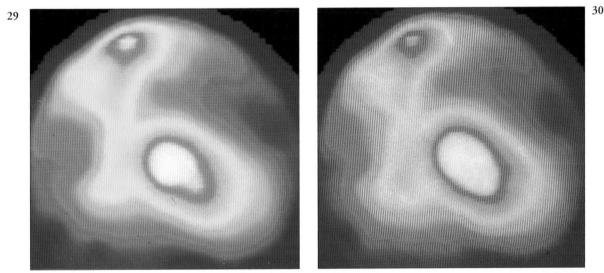

29 & 30 Nuclear techniques can define the impairment of ventricular contraction and occasionally demonstrate the aetiology of heart failure. A gated blood pool scan (systole, **29**; diastole, **30**) of a dilated poorly contracting left ventricle in heart failure.

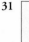

31

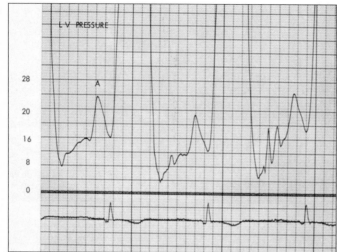

31–33 Haemodynamic monitoring will demonstrate the raised filling pressures characteristically found in heart failure as an increased left ventricular end-diastolic pressure (A) (**31**). The right atrial pressure may be raised and in atrial flutter will demonstrate characteristic flutter waves (F) (**32**) The increased right atrial pressure is observed clinically as a raised jugular venous pressure (see **22**). Increasing severity of left ventricular dysfunction may be evident as pulsus alternans (**33**). Compare with the non-invasive or indirect recording (**21**).

32

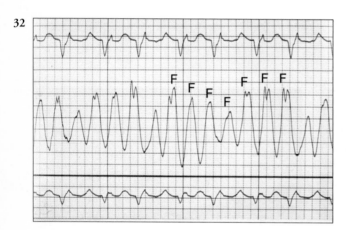

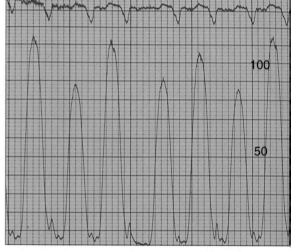

34

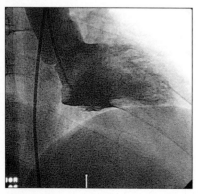

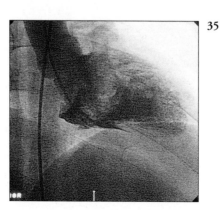

35

34 & 35 Contrast left ventriculography may be used to demonstrate a dilated ventricular cavity with poor contraction (systolic frame, **34**; diastolic frame, **35**). Coronary angiography may be useful in the assessment of the underlying cause of heart failure.

Causes of deterioration of heart failure

The aetiology of heart failure is dealt with in later sections, but it is important to recognize the precipitating causes of this condition. Many patients have well-compensated and stable heart failure but may develop much more severe symptoms due to an identified precipitating factor. The detection of such precipitating causes may have important therapeutic implications. In addition, patients with heart failure may have deterioration in their clinical state due to progression in the cause of the heart failure or to the onset of complications such as pulmonary or systemic embolism or arrhythmia.

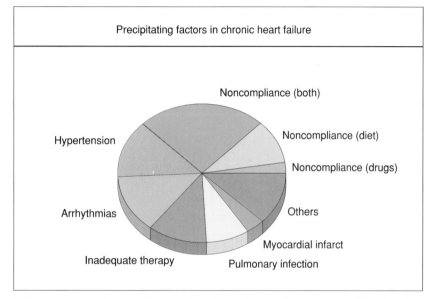

Precipitating factors in chronic heart failure

Noncompliance (both)

Noncompliance (diet)

Noncompliance (drugs)

Hypertension

Others

Arrhythmias

Myocardial infarct

Inadequate therapy

Pulmonary infection

36 Inappropriate reduction of therapy is probably the most frequent cause of deterioration. The use of a negatively inotropic drug such as a beta-blocker or antiarrhythmic agent may also lead to heart failure. Deterioration in the underlying cardiac condition may result in the onset of heart failure in a patient with stable cardiac disease. Others factors important in precipitating heart failure include systemic and cardiac infection (endocarditis is dealt with later), the development of a second form of heart disease such as myocardial infarction in a patient with valve disease or a further myocardial infarction in a patient with an impaired left ventricular function (Ghali *et al.,* 1988).

37
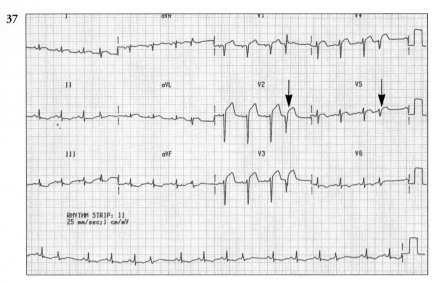

38
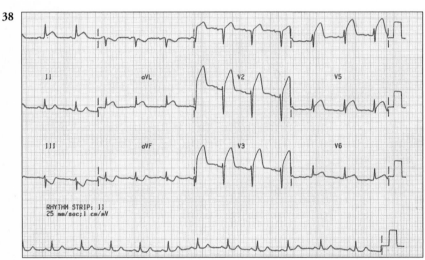

39
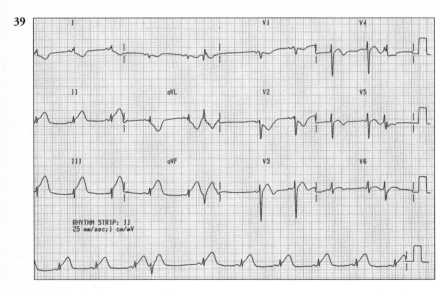

37–39 Electrocardiograms of a patient with an anterior myocardial infarction (**37**) showing sinus rhythm with atrial extrasystoles (arrows). There is ST segment elevation in V_{1-4} with lateral T wave inversion. Over the succeeding days, the patient developed further chest pain and extension of the anterior infarction as shown by further elevation of the anterior ST segments (**38**). ST segments are now elevated (V_{1-6}, I and AVL) with inferior ST depression (II, III and AVF). Subsequently, inferior ST segment elevation occurred (ST elevation in II, III and AVF with reciprocal changes in I, AVL, V_1 and V_2) which, due to the extent of myocardial damage, was accompanied by the development of acute left ventricular failure (**39**).

40–42 The development of tachyarrhythmias such as atrial fibrillation and flutter are common precipitating causes of heart failure. The change from sinus rhythm (**40**) to atrial flutter (**41**) (flutter waves are arrowed; there is 2:1 atrioventricular conduction) and fibrillation (**42**) in a patient with impaired left ventricular function due to an anterior myocardial infarction (ST segment elevation and Q waves V_{1-5}) led to the development of heart failure. Much less commonly, very persistent tachycardias may lead to failure in a normally functioning heart.

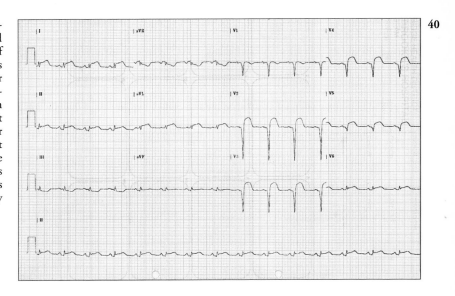

40

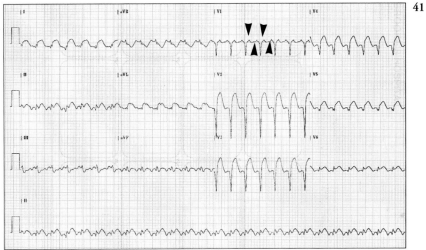

41

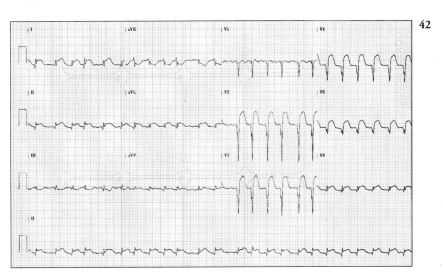

42

43

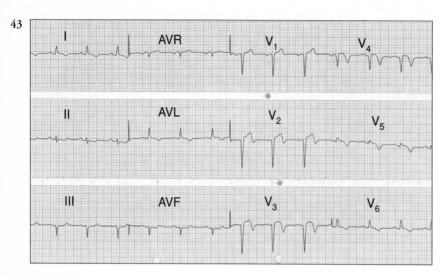

43 & 44 While ventricular arrhythmias are a common cause of sudden death in patients with heart failure, they may also precipitate heart failure. In this example, a patient with a known anterior left ventricular aneurysm (Q waves V_1–V_4 with ST elevation; **43**) presented with acute heart failure due to rapid ventricular tachycardia (broad complex, right bundle branch block with a positive deflection in AVR: atrioventricular dissociation is seen) (**44**).

44

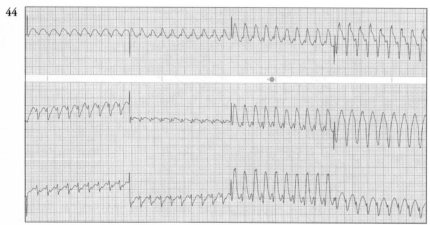

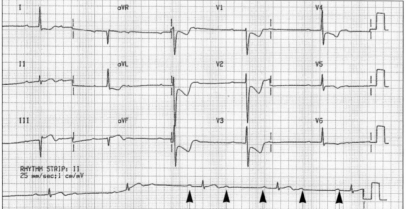

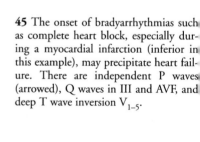

45 The onset of bradyarrhythmias such as complete heart block, especially during a myocardial infarction (inferior in this example), may precipitate heart failure. There are independent P waves (arrowed), Q waves in III and AVF, and deep T wave inversion $V_{1–5}$.

46–48 High output states may precipitate heart failure. Hyperthyroidism, shown here as left-sided exophthalmos and lid lag, is a common cause (**46**). Anaemia of whatever cause may exacerbate cardiac failure; shown here is iron deficiency anaemia with a smooth tongue and cheilitis (**47**). The cause of the anaemia is not usually evident clinically but occasionally superficial physical signs, as in this case with perioral haemangiomata indicative of hereditary haemorrhagic telangiectasia, indicate the potential presence of intra-abdominal bleeding (**48**).

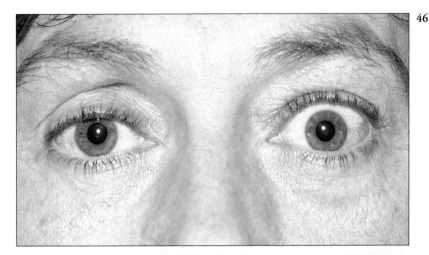

46

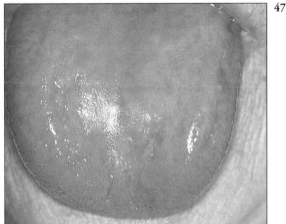

47

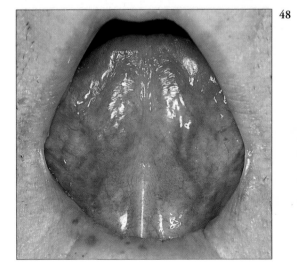

48

49 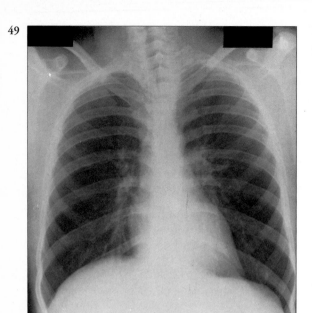 50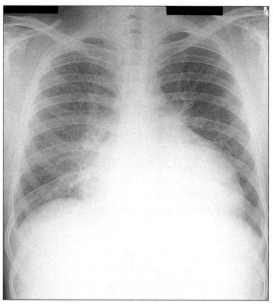

49 & 50 Chest radiograph in a patient before (**49**) and after (**50**) developing acute on chronic renal failure. The renal failure caused impairment of left ventricular function, development of the pericardial effusion and heart failure which is evident on the chest radiograph. Such changes are largely reversible using renal replacement therapy or transplantation.

Causes of heart failure

Causes of heart failure are legion as it may be the end-point of almost any form of cardiac disease. The commonest causes are coronary artery disease, valve disease, hyper-tension and cardiomyopathies. Congenital heart disease and a large number of rare abnormalities occasionally cause heart failure. The subsequent sections deal with the more commonly found forms of heart failure.

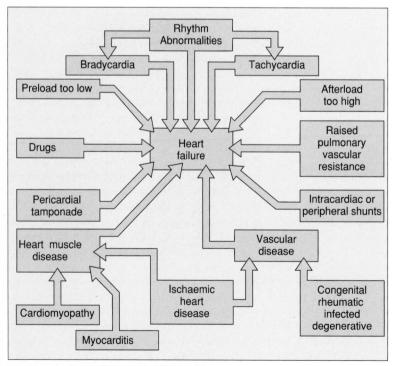

51 General scheme of the causes of heart failure.

Causes of heart failure
Coronary artery disease acute myocardial infarction, complications of infarction, chronic ischaemia.
Valvular heart disease
Heart muscle disease dilated cardiomyopathy, hypertrophic cardiomyopathy, restrictive cardio- myopathy, amyloidosis/sarcoidosis etc.
Hypertension
Pericardial disease
Congenital heart disease
Infection systemic and infective endocarditis, myocarditis rheumatic fever
Tachyarrhythmias
Cardiac tumours
Miscellaneous

52 Causes of heart failure.

2. CORONARY ARTERY DISEASE

Poor left ventricular function

Congestive heart failure is a not uncommon manifestation of coronary artery disease. Some patients will have sustained a previous myocardial infarction and in others the ischaemic area may have been replaced with a fibrous scar. The term 'ischaemic cardiomyopathy' has been used to describe a condition indistinguishable from dilated cardiomyopathy in which the cardiac symptoms of breathlessness and heart failure, rather than angina, are the predominant features. Recent observations suggest that in patients with coronary artery disease, anginal symptoms may be an insensitive indicator of recurrent myocardial ischaemia: such patients may develop heart failure caused by multiple ischaemic insults and diffuse ventricular fibrosis rather than a single discrete area of infarction or aneurysm.

The presence of ischaemia with coronary disease in patients with heart failure may have important therapeutic implications as in some, chronic ischaemia may be reversed by revascularization techniques such as PTCA or bypass grafting and lead to an improvement in ventricular function.

The commonest cause of heart failure in coronary artery disease is a reduction in normally contracting myocardium. However, the presence of mitral regurgitation due to papillary muscle dysfunction and left ventricular aneurysm formation are important causes of heart failure that may be treated surgically.

The presence of arrhythmias may exacerbate cardiac failure in coronary heart disease. Hypertensive and diabetic patients are particularly at risk of developing heart failure following myocardial infarction. The development of left ventricular failure after acute myocardial infarction is a poor prognostic feature.

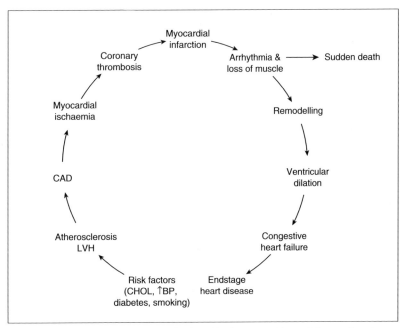

53 There is a sequence of events that leads to development of heart failure and end-stage heart disease and failure. This ring demonstrates the theoretical relationship between the development of heart failure and coronary risk factors such as hypercholesterolaemia, hypertension, diabetes and smoking. Coronary artery disease develops initially subclinically and then clinically. Myocardial infarction follows when the coronary thrombosis occurs in atherosclerotic arteries. With myocardial infarction there is loss of muscle, with potential arrhythmias and sudden death. Remodelling of the damaged left ventricle occurs, with ventricular dilatation leading in certain circumstances to heart failure.

54

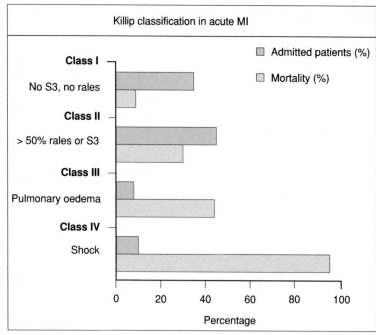

Killip classification in acute MI

☐ Admitted patients (%)

☐ Mortality (%)

Class I

No S3, no rales

Class II

> 50% rales or S3

Class III

Pulmonary oedema

Class IV

Shock

0   20   40   60   80   100

Percentage

55

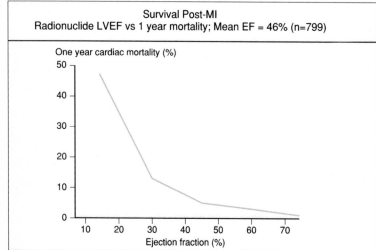

Survival Post-MI
Radionuclide LVEF vs 1 year mortality; Mean EF = 46% (n=799)

One year cardiac mortality (%)

50

40

30

20

10

0

10   20   30   40   50   60   70

Ejection fraction (%)

54 & 55 Extensive myocardial damage not only leads to the development of heart failure but also to a considerably increased cardiac mortality. In the short term, the signs of heart failure and shock are associated with very poor in-hospital survival. The long-term prognosis is also impaired and this is demonstrated in this graph of the relationship between left ventricular ejection fraction, as measured by gated blood pool scanning, and one-year cardiac mortality. Patients with a normal ejection fraction following myocardial infarction have an excellent one-year survival but as ejection fraction falls below 30 per cent, cardiac mortality rises steeply (Killip *et al.*, 1967, MPRG, 1983).

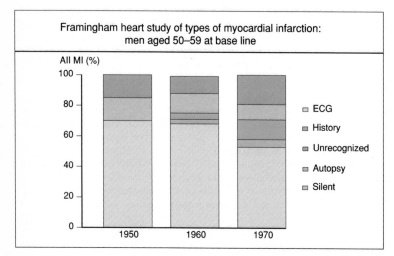

Framingham heart study of types of myocardial infarction:
men aged 50–59 at base line

All MI (%)

100

80

60

40

20

0

1950   1960   1970

☐ ECG

☐ History

☐ Unrecognized

☐ Autopsy

☐ Silent

56 While the majority of patients with myocardial infarction will present with the typical history, some will be silent and unrecognized (Sytkowski *et al.*, 1990).

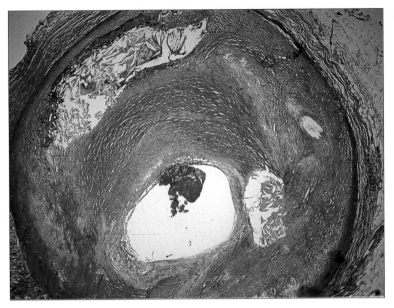

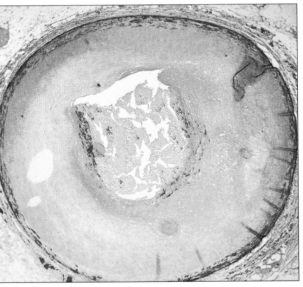

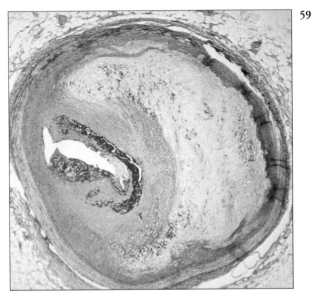

57–59 The mechanism of myocardial infarction is usually thrombotic occlusion of a stenosed coronary artery. There is disruption or fissuring of the superficial or deeper layers of the atherosclerotic plaque. Non-occlusive thrombus in a coronary artery which is already significantly narrowed (**57**). Occlusive thrombus consisting mainly of platelets in a left circumflex (**58**). Cross-section through a left anterior descending coronary artery at the site of thrombus (**59**). There is disruption of the superficial layer of the plaque and erythrocytes are seen below the surface.

60

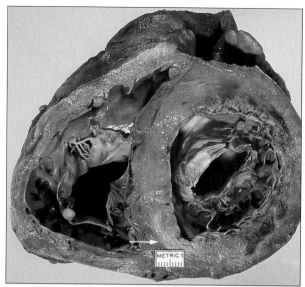

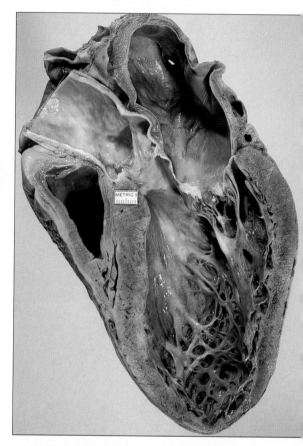

60–62 The development of heart failure following myocardial infarction may occur when there is one single extensive infarct or there is further damage to an already impaired left ventricle. Transverse section through the heart of a patient who died six days after an extensive lateral myocardial infarction (**60**). There is extensive necrosis in the anterior wall, the entire lateral wall and extending slightly in to the posterior wall. An old scar (arrow) is present in the ventricular septum which extends into the posterior wall. The left ventricular cavity is dilated. Extensive myocardial scarring with thinning of the ventricular wall especially at the apex, is shown (**61**). In long-standing heart failure following a myocardial infarction there may be compensating myocardial hypertrophy of the uninfarcted areas of ventricular wall. The transverse section through the heart of a 43-year-old man who had a two-year history of congestive heart failure is shown (**62**).There is a healed old posterior myocardial infarction seen as a dense white scar. The posterior wall is very thin but the remainder of the left ventricle has developed compensatory ventricular hypertrophy.

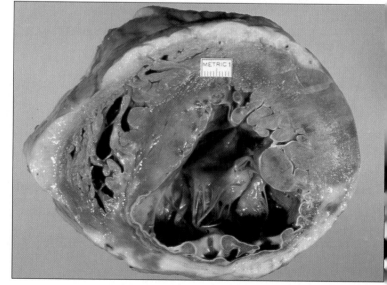

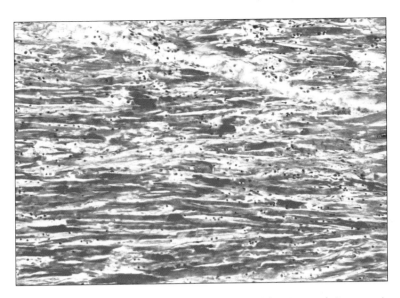

63 Histological section in acute myocardial infarction. There is coagulation necrosis with loss of cell nuclei and infiltration of polymorphonuclear leukocytes.

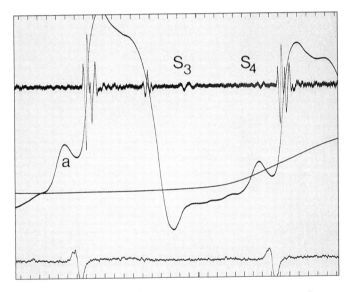

64 Examination of a patient with extensive left ventricular damage following acute myocardial infarction will reveal cardiomegaly and prominent *a* wave on the apex cardiogram (this may be felt). A third and fourth heart sound (S3 and S4) may be heard on auscultation.

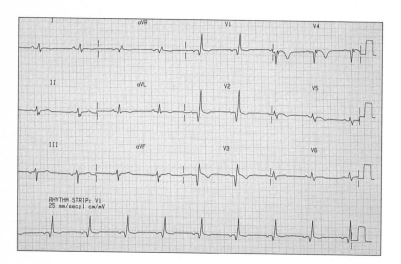

65 The electrocardiogram in heart failure due to extensive myocardial damage may often be non-specific; in this example there is an anterior infarction (Q waves V1–V5) with right bundle branch block (QR' in V1–V3. The development of bundle branch block following anterior myocardial infarction nearly always indicates widespread ventricular damage.

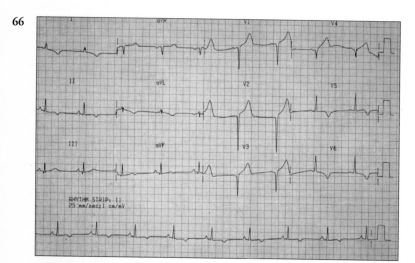

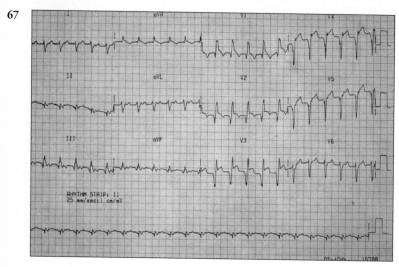

66 & 67 Arrhythmias in patients with acute myocardial infarction may lead to cardiac failure. The arrhythmias may be of supraventricular or ventricular origin. Shown here is a patient who has suffered an anterior myocardial infarction (ST elevation in V1–4 with Q in V1–4 and lateral T wave inversion) (**66**). Heart failure developed with the onset of a nodal tachycardia at a rate of approximately 150 beats per minute with right bundle branch block (**67**).

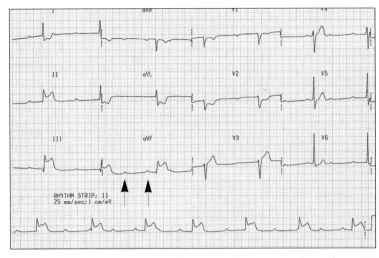

68 Bradycardia, in this case complete heart block, following an inferior myocardial infarction may lead to temporary heart failure. There are independent P waves (arrowed) with ST elevation in II, III and AVF.

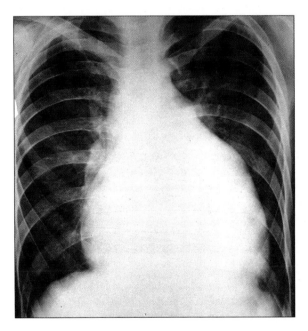

69 Chest radiograph showing a grossly enlarged heart following multiple myocardial infarctions. The radiological findings in heart failure may vary from a normally sized heart with pulmonary oedema to gross cardiac enlargement.

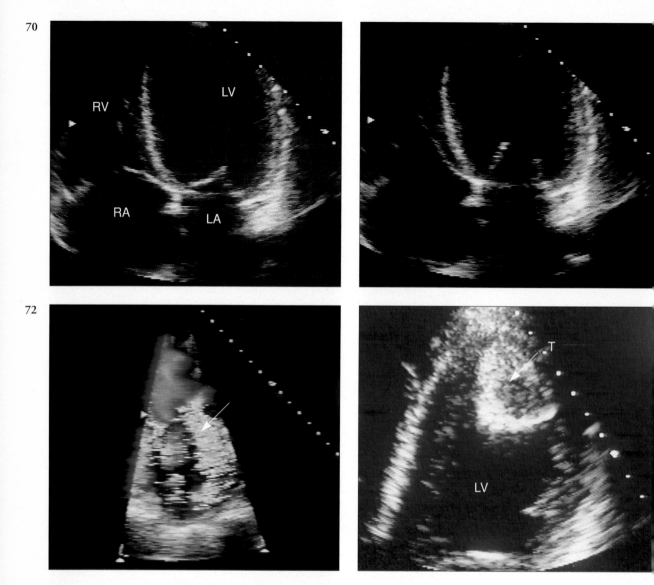

70–73 Echocardiography may be used to estimate left ventricular function in heart failure due to coronary heart disease as well as to diagnose the complications, especially in left ventricular thrombus and mitral regurgitation. Echocardiogram, apical long axis view (systole **70**, diastole **71**) showing left ventricular dilatation and poor contraction following an extensive myocardial infarction. Echocardiogram, apical long axis view, showing poor left ventricular function with a narrow jet of mild mitral regurgitation by colour flow Doppler; there is a turbulent (mosaic) area of colour from the mitral valve into the left atrium (arrowed) (**72**). Mild mitral regurgitation is a common accompaniment of poor left ventricular function due to abnormalities of the papillary muscles and mitral annular dilatation. Echocardiogram, apical long axis view, showing a left ventricular thrombus (T) at the apex following a myocardial infarction (**73**).

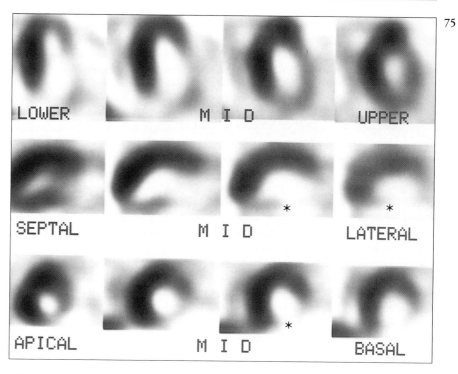

74 & 75 Myocardial perfusion scanning may be useful for defining the presence and extent of fixed and reversible defects on exercise. Shown here is a tomographic MIBI scintigram with inferior perfusion defects (fixed) at rest (**74**) due to inferior previous myocardial infarction (arrowed), and further reversible defects on exercise (∗) (**75**).

76

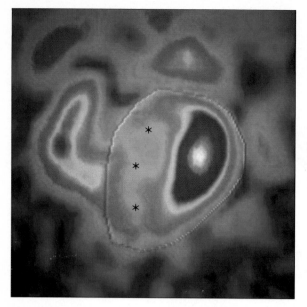

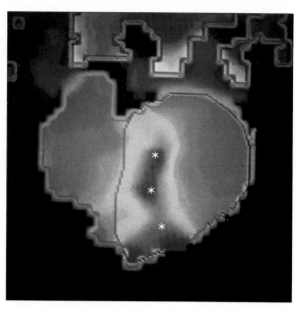

76 & 77 Gated blood pool scan in a patient who has an anterior myocardial infarction due to occlusion of the left anterior descending coronary artery. The amplitude image (**76**) and phase image (**77**) indicate an akinetic anterior wall (∗).

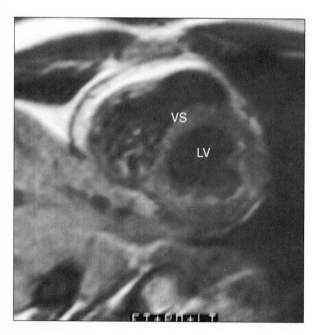

78 Magnetic resonance scan, left ventricle short axis view, in a patient with ischaemic heart disease. The ventricular cavity is slightly dilated and the septum thinned (VS).

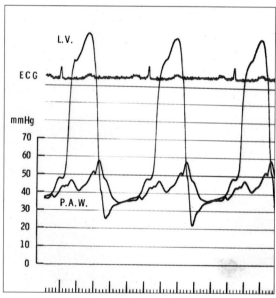

79 Haemodynamic tracing showing a markedly elevated (twice normal) left ventricular, end-diastolic and pulmonary wedge pressure (PAW).

80a
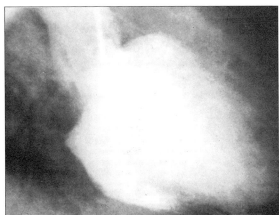
80b
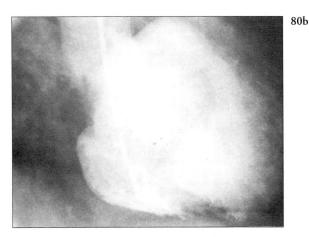

80a & 80b A left ventricular angiogram (systole, **80a**; diastole, **80b**). The left ventricular function is extremely poor.

Mitral regurgitation

An early complication of acute myocardial infarction, acute severe mitral regurgitation, may occur during the course of a myocardial infarction because of rupture of all or part of a papillary muscle. Papillary muscle ischaemia or fibrosis may lead to dysfunction of the mitral subvalvular apparatus and subsequent chronic mitral regurgitation. In addition, dilatation of the mitral annulus may also cause mitral regurgitation. The development of mitral regurgitation following acute myocardial infarction is frequently associated with cardiac failure. The commonest location of sites for myocardial infarction is inferior, but the amount of myocardial damage may be limited to only affecting the papillary muscle or the surrounding area.

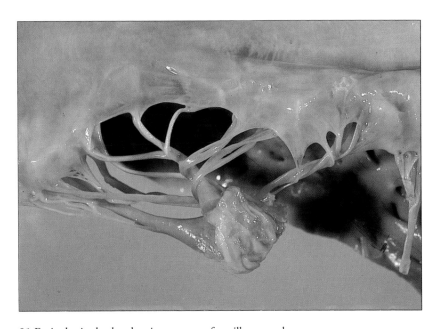

81 Excised mitral valve showing rupture of papillary muscle.

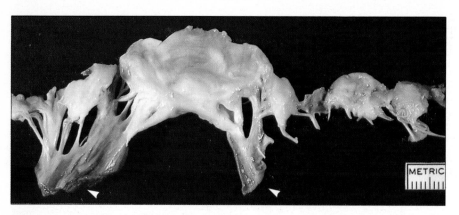

82 Excised mitral valve showing ischaemic scarring of the papillary muscle (arrows).

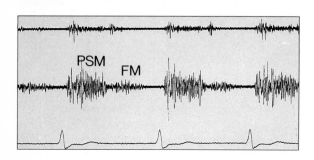

83 Phonocardiogram of severe mitral regurgitation showing a loud pansystolic murmur (PSM) with a diastolic flow murmur (FM) and a third heart sound (S3) (on the upper trace).

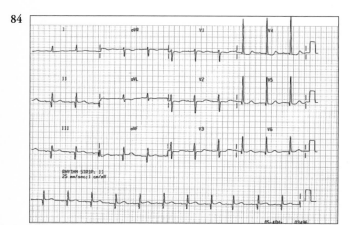

84

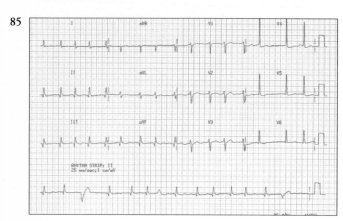

85

84 & 85 Electrocardiogram showing an inferior myocardial infarction (Q waves in II, III and AVF) in sinus rhythm (**84**). This myocardial infarction led to severe mitral regurgitation and with the onset of atrial fibrillation (**85**) heart failure ensued.

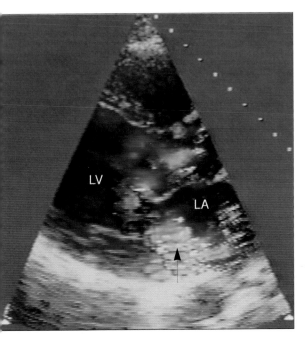
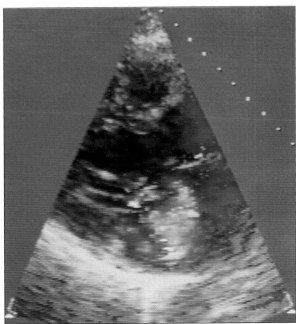

86 & 87 Cross-sectional echocardiograms, parasternal long axis view (early systole, **86**; late systole, **87**), showing mitral regurgitation as a jet of mosaic colour flow Doppler (arrow) arising from the prolapsing mitral valve and entering a normally sized left atrium (LA). Left ventricular (LV) function is only moderately impaired.

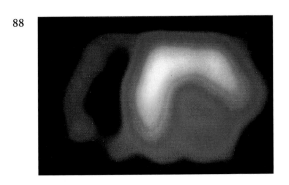
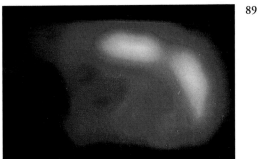
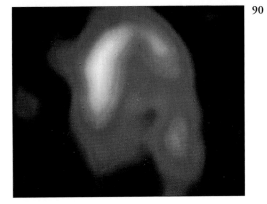

88–90 Thallium tomographic scans (short axis view, **88**; vertical long axis view, **89**; horizontal long axis view, **90**) showing a fixed perfusion defect involving the inferior and lateral walls of the left ventricle. Involvement of this area of the left ventricular wall may lead to mitral regurgitation.

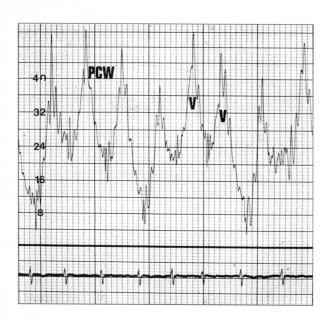

91 Haemodynamic tracing in mitral regurgitation following acute myocardial infarction. There is a high *v* or systolic wave in the pulmonary capillary wedge pressure (PCW).

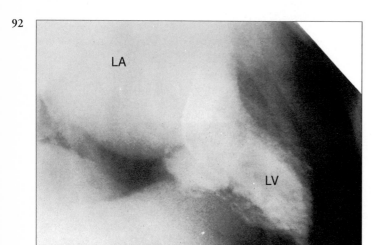

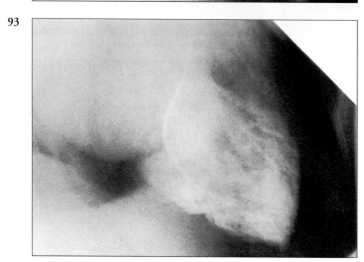

92 & 93 Left ventricular angiogram (systole, **92**; diastole, **93**) showing inferior dyskinesia and gross mitral regurgitation due to papillary muscle dysfunction. The overall left ventricular function is well preserved.

Ventricular septal defect

Ventricular septal defect is an uncommon but well recognized early complication of acute myocardial infarction. Usually the defects are large and rapidly lead to the onset of heart failure and a low output state. Most commonly, ventricular septal defects occur in anterior infarctions though they may be inferior, in which case the mortality rate is greater. Clinically, it may be difficult to differentiate mitral regurgitation from a ventricular septal defect but echocardiography can readily enable a diagnosis to be made at the bedside.

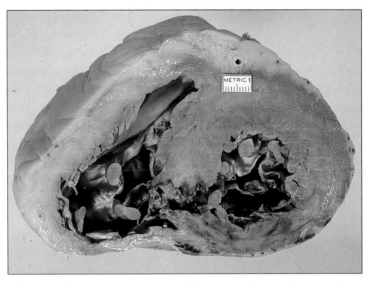

94 Section through the posterior part of the septum showing a large ventricular septal defect that occurred secondary to an acute myocardial infarction.

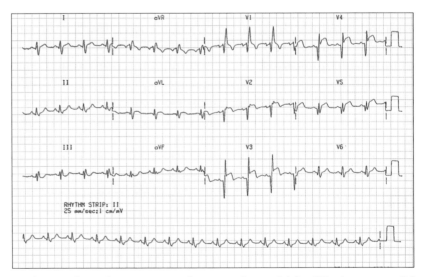

95 Electrocardiography in a patient with a ventricular septal defect following a myocardial infarction usually shows an anteroseptal myocardial infarction (Q waves V1–V5), in this case with right bundle branch block (RSR' in V1).

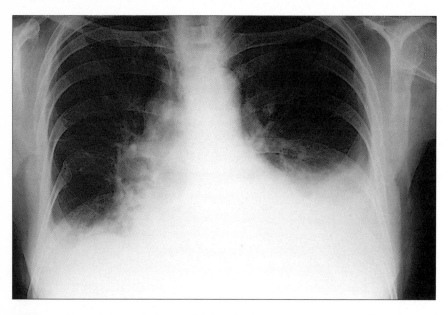

96 Chest radiograph in ventricular septal defect showing pulmonary plethora, bilateral pleural effusions and an enlarged heart.

97   98   99

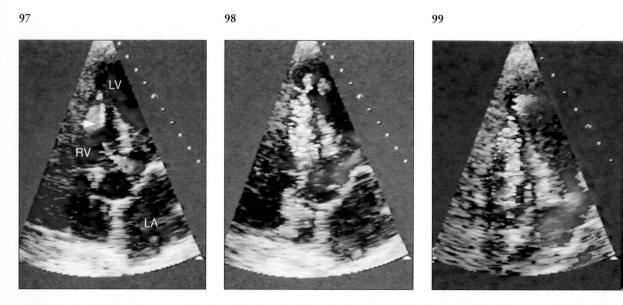

97–99 A series of echocardiograms with colour flow Doppler, four chamber view, which show a jet of turbulent (mosaic) blood flow through the muscular portion of the septum (arrowed). As the cardiac cycle progresses, this abnormal, turbulent jet passes through the right ventricle towards the tricuspid valve. Echocardiography shows the septal defect in an area of akinetic muscle but the defect is often rather ragged in appearance and there may be malalignment of the edges.

100 Left ventricular angiogram in the left anterior oblique projection showing contrast filling the left ventricle and spilling across the ventricular septal defect into the right ventricle.

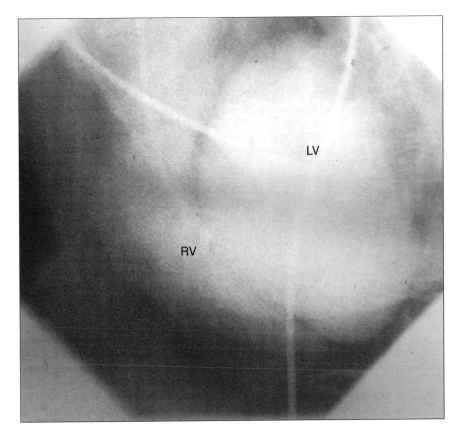

Left ventricular aneurysm

Left ventricular aneurysm, which is a late complication of myocardial infarction, may be defined as the systolic expansion (paradoxical or dyskinetic) of a portion of the left ventricular wall. This most commonly occurs in the antero-apical segments and consists largely of scar tissue. Dyskinetic segments produce a mechanical disadvantage by a combination of systolic expansion and the loss of effective contraction. A true aneurysm has a wide mouth, in contrast to the narrow entrance point of a false or pseudo-aneurysm, which represents a well-defined, localized myocardial rupture. The haemorrhage which occurs through this rupture is limited by pericardial adhesions. Left ventricular aneurysm formation may occur following cardiac trauma but the vast majority of patients have underlying coronary artery disease with prior myocardial infarction. Most commonly, aneurysms occur with total occlusion of the subtending coronary artery (usually left anterior descending) with a poor collateral blood flow. The frequency of left ventricular aneurysm after myocardial infarction depends on the incidence of transmural

myocardial infarction. Approximately half the patients with large aneurysms present with symptoms of heart failure with or without angina; one-third present with angina alone and 10–15 per cent with ventricular arrhythmias. While ventricular aneurysms are often filled with thrombus, embolic events occur relatively infrequently, usually some time after the infarction. Heart failure due to left ventricular aneurysm may occur weeks, months or even, occasionally, years after an acute myocardial infarction. The detection of a left ventricular aneurysm is important in patients with heart failure, as in some it may be successfully treated by surgical resection, if it is well demarcated and the remaining left ventricular function is adequately preserved. Classically, an anterior praecordial bulge may be felt and a third heart sound heard. Persistent ST segment elevation is often present on the electrocardiogram. Cardiac arrhythmias, particularly ventricular tachycardia, may precipitate heart failure in a patient with left ventricular aneurysm. Diagnosis is best made using magnetic resonance imaging or left ventricular angiography.

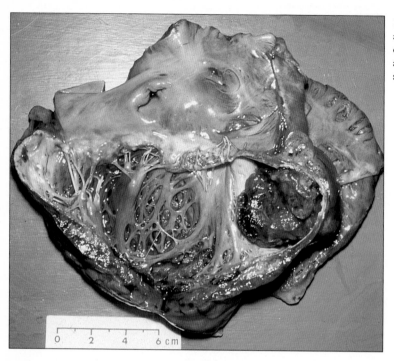

101 Pathological specimen from a patient with an antero-apical myocardial infarction who developed a left ventricular aneurysm. A thinned area of the apex overlying the thrombus is clearly seen.

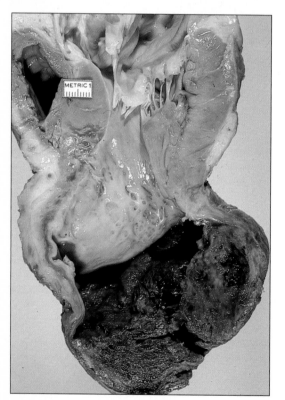

102 Pathological specimen cut in an echocardiographic long axis section of huge left ventricular aneurysm filled with laminated thrombus.

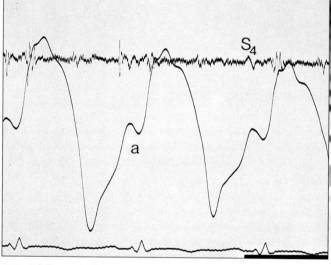

103 A left ventricular aneurysm may be suggested clinically from the presence of a very tall *a* wave (representing 50 per cent of the overall apical displacement, here shown on an indirect recording) together with late systolic motion. The dyskinetic segment may also be felt in the anterior chest.

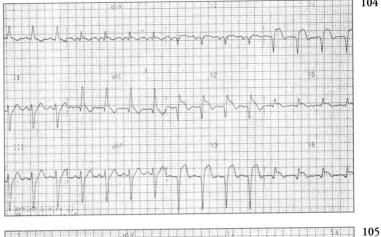

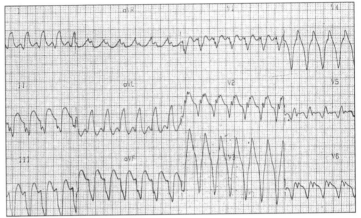

104 & 105 Electrocardiogram with persistent praecordial ST segment elevation in a patient with antero-apical left ventricular aneurysm (**104**). Subsequently, this patient developed ventricular tachycardia (**105**).

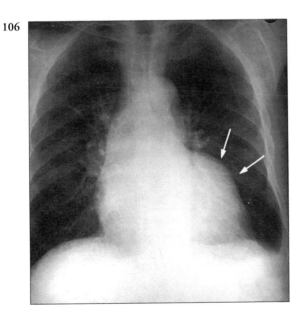

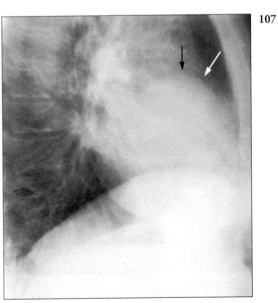

106 & 107 Chest radiographs (posterior–anterior projection, **106**; lateral projection, **107**) showing a bulge (arrows) on the left ventricular border of the heart which is anterior on the lateral view due to a left aneurysm.

108a

An

LV

109

111

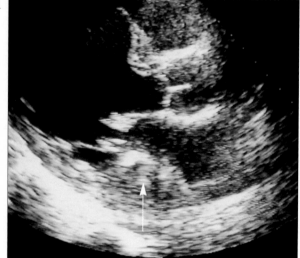

108a–111 Cross-sectional echocardiogram, apical long axis view, of an apical left ventricular aneurysm. Echocardiography may show an akinetic segment, particularly if filled by thrombus, but is rather limited in the examination of the apex which is the most frequent site of aneurysm formation. The dyskinetic and bulging apical segment (An) may be visualized (systole, **108a**; diastole, **108b**); the echocardiogram also allows examination of the size and function of the base of the ventricle, which may determine the suitability for surgery. Left ventricular thrombus often overlies areas of aneurysm formation especially at the apex (arrow) (**109**) and the whole sac may become almost obliterated by clot (arrow) (**110**), here shown in a parasternal long axis view with an anterior septal clot-filled aneurysm. Echocardiography may distinguish a true from a false aneurysm; here an expansile filling defect is seen behind the left atrium, which originates from a free wall rupture (arrow) (**111**).

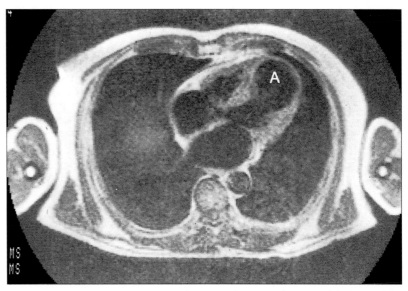

112 Magnetic resonance image, sagittal section, showing a thin area of the apex of the left ventricle due to an aneurysm (A).

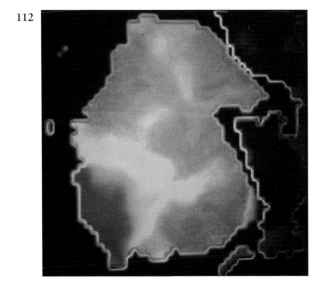

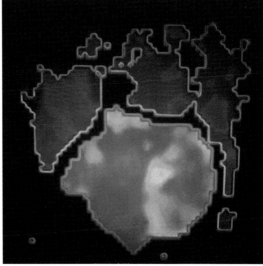

113 & 114 Gated blood pool imaging in left ventricular aneurysm (pre-operative, **113**; post-operative after resection of the aneurysm, **114**). These are amplitude images and a large area of the apex is not contracting (dark red on the image). After resection of the aneurysm, this area of akinesis is no longer evident.

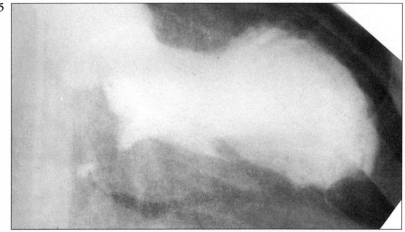

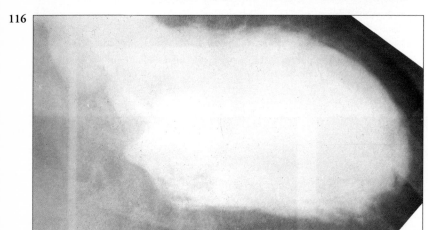

115 & 116 Left ventricular angiogram (systole, **115**; diastole, **116**) showing a large antero-apical left ventricular aneurysm evident on the systolic frame.

Right ventricular infarction

Most patients who develop heart failure following a myocardial infarction will do so due to the extent of left ventricular damage. However, a small proportion of patients will develop a low cardiac state without pulmonary oedema due to right ventricular infarction. This does not usually occur alone but in association with left ventricular infarction either inferiorly or, less frequently, anteriorly. The classical haemodynamic situation is a patient with low cardiac output, in shock, who has a low pulmonary wedge pressure and a high right atrial filling pressure. The diagnosis may be obtained by electrocardiography, echocardiography or gated blood pool scanning.

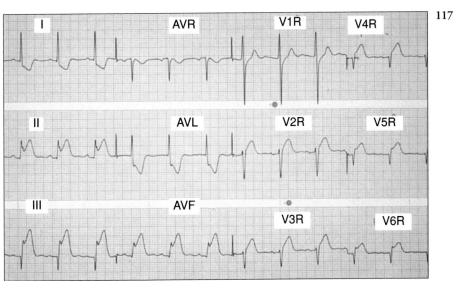

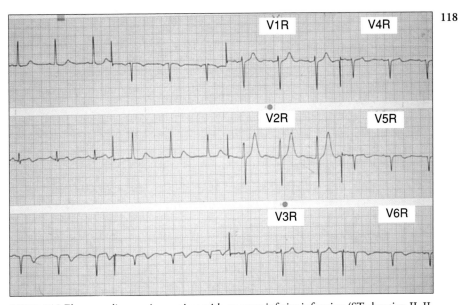

117 & 118 Electrocardiogram in a patient with an acute inferior infarction (ST elevation II, II, AVF) who presented with low cardiac output (**117**). Right-sided chest leads show ST segment elevation (V2R–V6R). Two days later, the electrocardiogram shows only the inferior infarction which has evolved to Q waves without persistent ST segment elevation in the right-sided leads (**118**).

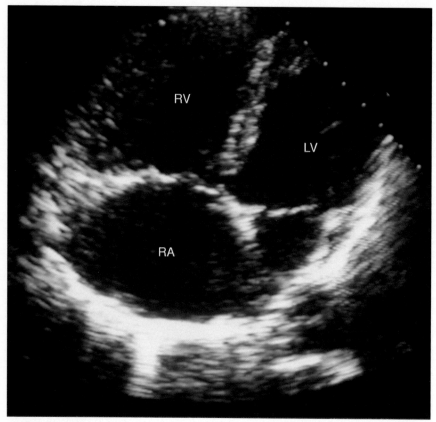

119 In patients with right ventricular infarction, echocardiography shows a dilated right ventricle with accompanying regional wall motion abnormality of the left ventricle.

3. Valvular Heart Disease

Chronic mitral valve disease

Heart failure may develop in the presence of mitral valve disease of all types. Rheumatic heart disease may result in mitral stenosis and regurgitation although isolated regurgitation is usually non-rheumatic in origin. Mitral stenosis, when severe, will cause a low output state and heart failure in the presence of a small heart with left atrial enlargement. The development of shortness of breath and heart failure is often insidious and the clinical diagnosis is best confirmed using echocardiography. A floppy mitral valve is a very common finding and usually causes no symptoms. Only when the regurgitation is severe, and particularly in the presence of ruptured chordae tendinae, mitral annular dilatation and impaired left ventricular contraction, will heart failure ensue. Ruptured chordae may present acutely or with progressive breathlessness and heart failure. The diagnosis is made using echocardiography. Ischaemia and infarction due to coronary artery disease may involve the papillary muscles, and there are many other causes of mitral regurgitation but all are much less common.

Rheumatic fever

Rheumatic fever is the delayed non-suppurative sequela of a pharyngeal infection with a group A streptococcus. There has been a marked decline in the incidence of rheumatic fever in the West in the last few decades; the reason for this is unclear but there does seem to be have been a recent recurrence. Rheumatic heart disease still constitutes a major cause of death from heart disease in younger patients in the developing parts of the world. Patients may present with an erythema marginatum, subcutaneous nodules, chorea and rheumatic pneumonitis. Cardiac lesions include pericarditis, myocarditis, conduction system disease and endocarditis. Mitral regurgitation occurs early and mitral stenosis and aortic involvement later. Less frequently, other valvular disease may occur. Heart failure may occur early due to myocardial involvement or later due to valvular disease.

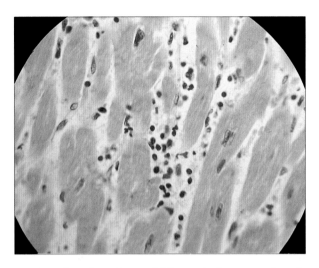

120 Histological specimen of left ventricular myocardium in rheumatic fever. The myocardium is infiltrated by lymphocytes during the acute phase of the disease.

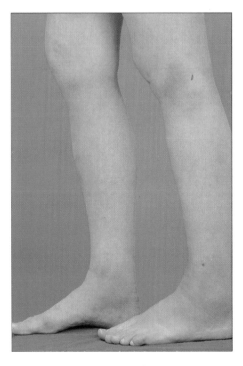

121 Clinically, rheumatic fever presents with swollen, tender joints as shown here.

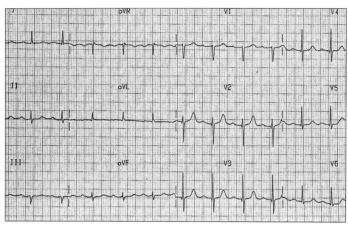

122 The electrocardiogram is non-specific and will often show first degree heart block (PR interval exceeds 220ms).

123   124   125

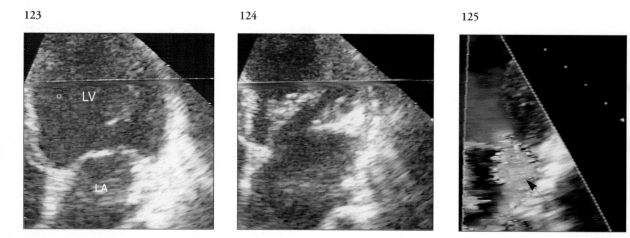

123–125 The echocardiogram in acute rheumatic fever shows a thickened and deformed mitral valve (systole, **123**; diastole, **124**) with predominant regurgitation (arrow) showing a turbulent regurgitative jet (colour flow Doppler, **125**); with progressive healing, the valves become predominantly stenosed.

Mitral stenosis

Approximately a quarter of all patients with rheumatic heart disease have pure mitral stenosis and more than a third have combined mitral stenosis and regurgitation. Rheumatic mitral valve disease predominantly occurs in women. The most frequent pathological feature in rheumatic involvement of the mitral valve is fusion of the mitral commissures, cusps and subvalve apparatus. The typical stenotic valve is often funnel-shaped and is described as a fish mouth or buttonhole. Usually, severe mitral stenosis follows the development of rheumatic fever by some years. The normal mitral valve orifice in adults is 4–6 cm; when this is reduced towards or below 1 cm, the diagnosis of severe mitral stenosis can be made. Mitral obstruction leads to elevated left atrial and pulmonary venous and capillary pressures. Pulmonary congestion leads to breathlessness, initially on exercise but latterly at rest. A deterioration of exercise tolerance or heart failure frequently occurs with the onset of atrial fibrillation, as loss of atrial contraction substantially reduces cardiac output. Chest pain, thromboembolism and infective endocarditis may all be presenting features of rheumatic mitral disease. Diagnosis can usually be made by clinical examination and confirmed by electrocardiography. Doppler ultrasound can be used to measure the mitral valve orifice. The differential diagnosis of thematic mitral stenosis includes other causes of mitral valve obstruction such as left atrial tumour and congenital mitral stenosis.

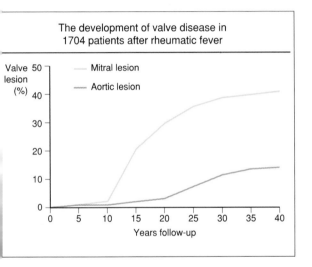

126 Following rheumatic fever, approximately 40 per cent of a sample of 1,704 patients in Dusseldorf developed mitral valve disease. This usually started some ten years after the initial event and compares to the lesser involvement and slower development of aortic disease (Horstkotte *et al.*, 1991).

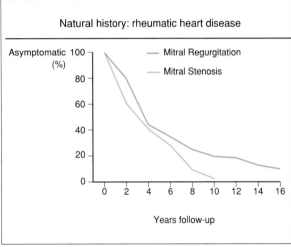

127 During follow-up, patients with rheumatic mitral stenosis become symptomatic earlier than those with predominant regurgitation (Horstkotte *et al.*, 1991).

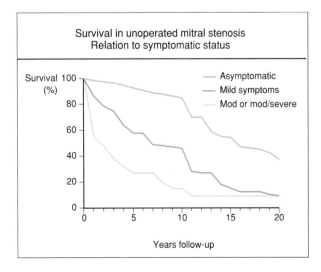

128 Life table analysis of survival in unoperated patients with mitral stenosis. Asymptomatic patients have 40 per cent 20-year survival whereas those with more severe symptoms have a much more restricted prognosis (Rowe *et al.*, 1960).

129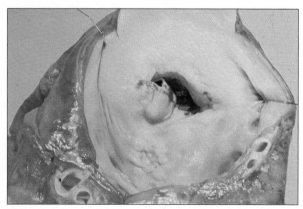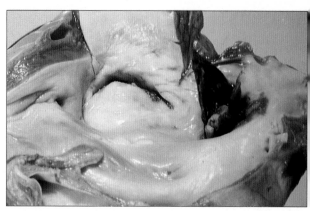

129 & 130 Pathology of mitral valve stenosis viewed from the left atrium. A narrowed and thickened valve is seen with marked commissural fusion (**129**). A typical fish mouth appearance of the mitral valve with thrombus lying within the left atrial appendage (**130**).

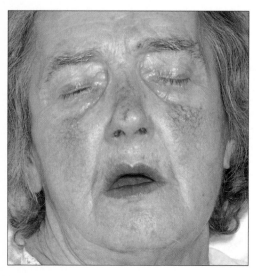

131 Typical malar flush of mitral stenosis. This is a non-specific finding due to low cardiac output.

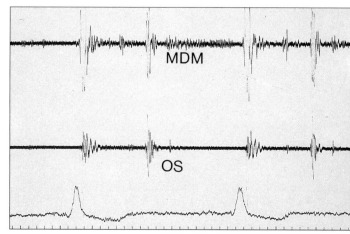

133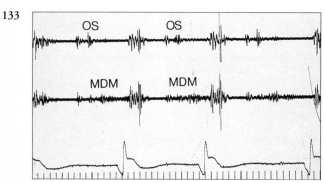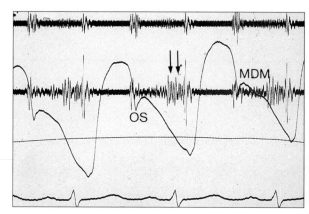

132–134 The murmur of mitral stenosis is characteristically a mid-diastolic rumble best heard at the apex with the bell of the stethoscope. The physical signs are demonstrated here by a series of phonocardiograms. In mild mitral obstruction, the mid-diastolic murmur (MDM) is best heard with the patient lying on the left side and may require exercise to accentuate it (**132**). With increasing severity of mitral obstruction, the murmur becomes longer and louder, starting earlier in diastole (**133**). If the patient is in sinus rhythm, then a pre-systolic murmur may be heard (arrows) which follows an opening snap and a long diastolic murmur (**134**).

135 & 136 The electrocardiogram in mitral stenosis most commonly shows left atrial enlargement (biphasic P wave in V1) and signs of right ventricular hypertrophy due to secondary pulmonary hypertension. Left ventricular hypertrophy may also be present as in this example due to mitral stenosis and regurgitation (**135**). Heart failure or pulmonary hypertension may develop without electrocardiographic right ventricular hypertrophy. With the onset of atrial fibrillation or flutter as in this example (**136**), heart failure may ensue.

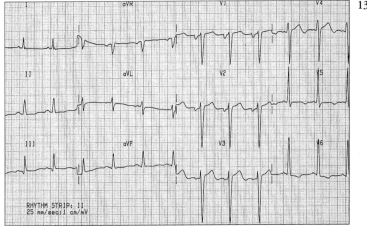

135

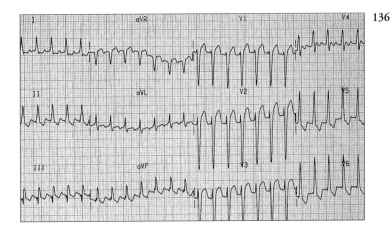

136

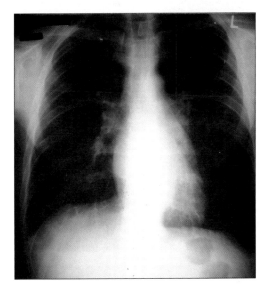

137 Chest radiograph in mitral stenosis with an enlarged left atrium and appendage without overall enlargement of cardiac silhouette. On this penetrated film, pulmonary venous congestion is not seen but pulmonary oedema may occur, in particular, with the onset of atrial fibrillation.

138

140

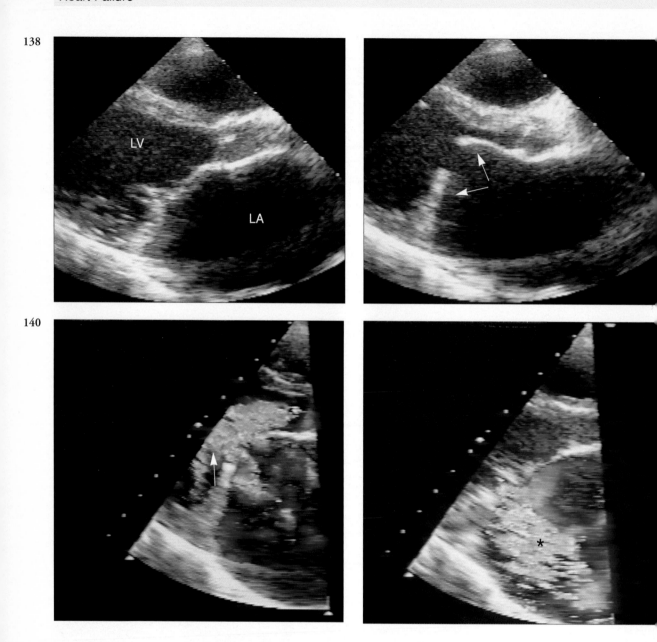

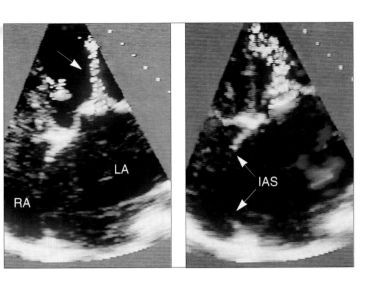

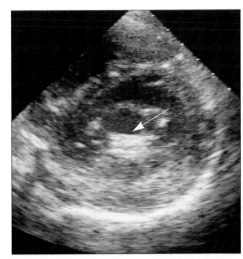

143

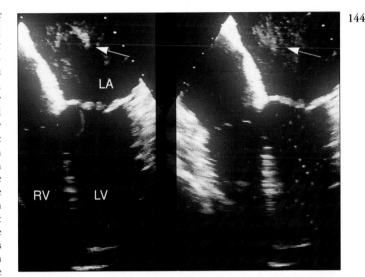

144

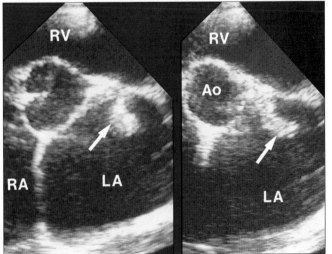

145

138–145 The echocardiogram is the diagnostic method of choice for determining the presence and severity of mitral valve disease and its associated complications including left atrial enlargement and thrombus formation. Echocardiogram, parasternal long axis view, in mitral stenosis showing in systole (**138**) the thickened mitral valve which domes in diastole (**139**) (arrows). Colour flow Doppler imaging may demonstrate the obstruction to the mitral valve and allow the documentation of its severity by continuous wave Doppler. In the same patient, a diastolic frame shows a turbulent or mosaic forward jet (arrow) in the left ventricle (**140**) and a regurgitant jet into the atrium in early systole (∗) (**141**). Two diastolic frames from the apical long axis view (**142**) show the candle flame shape (arrows) and movement of the forward jet: on the left, an early diastolic frame shows a narrow turbulent or mosaic jet across the mitral valve extending towards the apex from the mitral valve. Later on in diastole, the jet widens. In this example, severe mitral stenosis is associated with considerable large atrial enlargement with bowing of the interatrial septum (IAS) towards the right atrium. The mitral valve can be imaged and the orifice measured directly (arrow) in a parasternal short axis view, although this method of assessment tends to underestimate the severity of obstruction (**143**). The initial development of left atrial thrombus usually occurs in the left atrial appendage and is often associated with atrial blood stasis which can be demonstrated by spontaneous echo contrast. In this example on a transoesophageal four chamber view in a patient with mitral stenosis, a swirling pattern of echo contrast is seen (arrow) (**144**). While transoesophageal echocardiography is the method of choice for imaging the appendage directly, the thrombus can be seen on transthoracic echo when it emerges from the appendage. The movement of a pedunculated thrombus in the left atrium arising from the appendage is shown in two frames of parasternal short axis view (**145**).

146

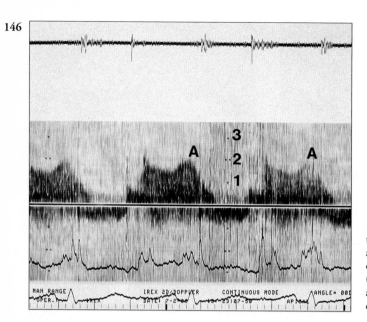

146 & 147 Doppler ultrasound allows the assessment of the transmitral gradient and calculations of the mitral orifice area. In sinus rhythm, the increased transvalvular velocity can be seen (in this example 2 m/s) (146). A large atrial peak (A) is observed. Following the onset of atrial fibrillation, the atrial peak is lost and a varying length of the cardiac cycle can be seen (147).

147

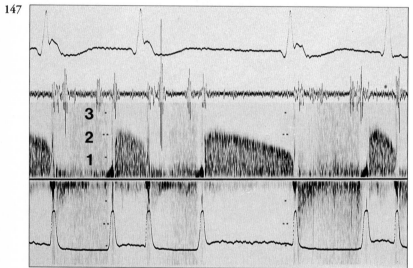

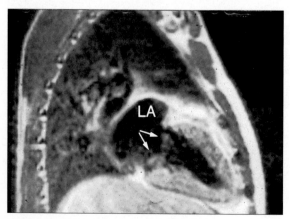

148 Magnetic resonance imaging, sagittal section, showing a thick mitral valve (arrows) and an enlarged left atrium (LA).

Mitral balloon valvuloplasty

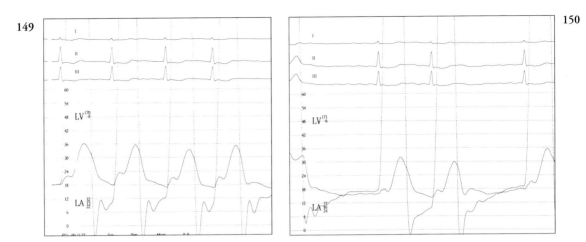

149   150

Haemodynamic tracing in mitral stenosis in atrial fibrillation. There is a resting gradient between the left atrial (measured directly by transeptal puncture) and the left ventricular end-diastolic pressure (LVEDP) (**149**). Following mitral balloon valvotomy, the gradient at end-diastole across the valve is abolished (**150**).

151–157 A significantly stenotic mitral valve (area >1 cm^2) which is mobile or pliable without significant regurgitation and sub-valvular fusion or calcification may be successfully treated by valvuloplasty. While the closed operation without cardiopulmonary bypass is no longer used in the West, it is frequently performed in countries with less access to advanced medical technology. Percutaneous balloon dilatation may produce a similar result. Left ventricular angiogram in right anterior oblique projection (systole, **151**; diastole, **152**) showing a thickened domed mitral valve (arrows). Such appearances would suggest a suitable valve for balloon dilatation. A sequence of films shows an Inoue valvuloplasty balloon passed from the right to left atrium by transeptal puncture. The balloon is partly across the inter-atrial septum in its stretched position (arrow) on a coiled guide wire (*) (**153**). The stretching tube and guide are removed and the balloon is seen partly inflated in the left atrium (**154**). The balloon is shown partly inflated through the mitral orifice (**155**, over page) in right anterior oblique projection. The balloon is progressively inflated until the stenotic valve is caught in its waist (arrows) (**156,** over page) and finally the balloon is fully inflated to a predetermined size to achieve commissural splitting (**157**, over page).

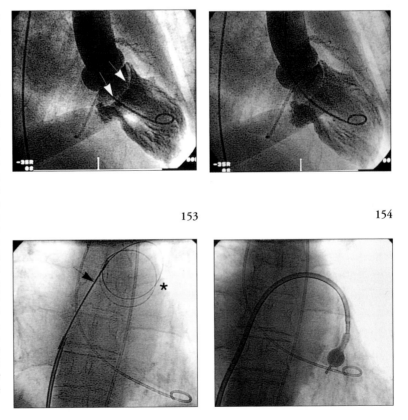

151   152

153   154

155

156

157

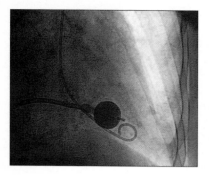 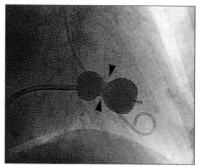 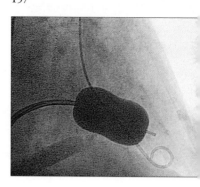

Mitral valve regurgitation

Mitral valve prolapse is a disease of very diverse clinical presentation; most cases have simply the murmur and/or click associated with this condition. The other end of the clinical spectrum includes patients who become symptomatic with severe mitral regurgitation. While the mild form predominates in younger women, the severe form with mitral regurgitation is more common in men. Mitral regurgitation, especially in a mild form, may be associated with a large number of systemic diseases such as Marfan's syndrome, Ehlers–Danlos syndrome and pseudoxanthoma elasticum. Myxomatous changes in the mitral valve suggest an abnormality of collagen is probably responsible. Degeneration within the central core of the chordae tendinae leads to chordae rupture and the progression from mild to severe regurgitation. Myxomatous changes in the mitral annulus may lead to annular dilatation and calcification which may increase the severity of valvular regurgitation. Symptoms in chronic mitral regurgitation may be related to

the severity of valvular leak and its rate of progression, pulmonary hypertension and the presence of other heart disease. Embolization and pulmonary oedema are less common in mitral regurgitation than in mitral stenosis. Patients with severe mitral regurgitation of chronic onset have a greatly enlarged left atrium and are limited by fatigue and low cardiac output. Right heart failure may be a prominent feature. Acute mitral regurgitation usually occurs due to rupture of chordae tendinae which may be due to chordal degeneration or endocarditis and may produce acute pulmonary oedema. Investigation of patients with mitral regurgitation is directed towards the cause of the valve abnormality, its severity and its effect on left ventricular function and pulmonary artery pressure. This can usually be carried out non-invasively using echocardiography, and Doppler and magnetic resonance scanning, but left ventriculography is often required to assess the severity of regurgitation.

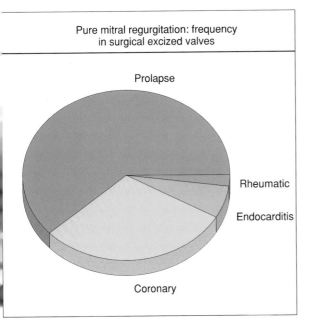

Pure mitral regurgitation: frequency
in surgical excized valves

Prolapse

Rheumatic

Endocarditis

Coronary

158 Frequency distribution of causes of pure mitral regurgitation in surgically excised valves. While there are a large number of causes of mild mitral regurgitation, the commonest causes of severe regurgitation are mitral valve prolapse, coronary disease and endocarditis (Waller *et al.*, 1982).

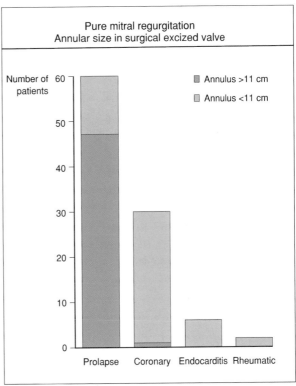

Pure mitral regurgitation
Annular size in surgical excized valve

Number of patients

■ Annulus >11 cm
□ Annulus <11 cm

Prolapse Coronary Endocarditis Rheumatic

159 Dilatation of the mitral annulus is frequently present in mitral prolapse. This is much less common in other causes of mitral regurgitation requiring surgery (Waller *et al.*, 1982).

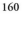

160

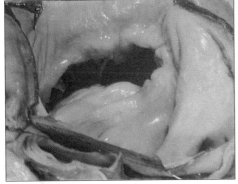

161

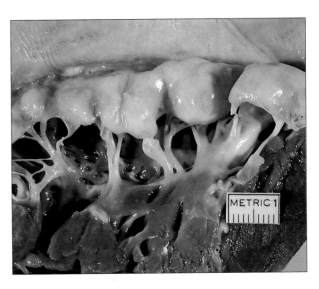

160 & 161 Pathological features of non-rheumatic mitral regurgitation. The valve is viewed from the opened left atrium and has a scalloped and redundant appearance. The orifice is of normal size (**160**). The surface area of the valve is increased, producing the scalloped appearance with focal fibrous thickening of the leaflets and thickened chordae tendinae (**161**).

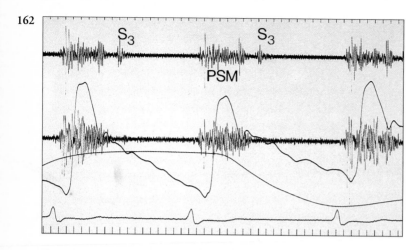

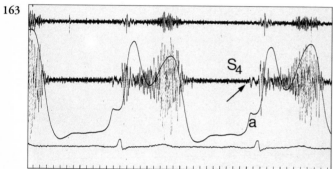

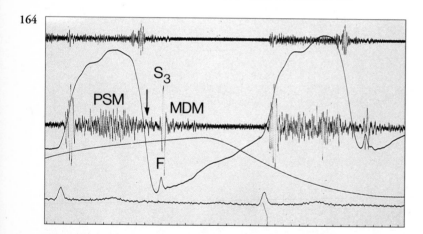

162–164 A series of phonocardiograms and indirect pulse and apex recordings which demonstrate the physical signs in mitral regurgitation. The pulse in significant mitral regurgitation is characteristically brisk and ill-sustained (**162**). The apical impulse becomes sustained and there is a palpable fourth heart sound (S_4 and a wave on the apical trace) (**163**). The murmur of mitral regurgitation is pansystolic (**162**) though may be accentuated in late systole (**163**). Third and fourth heart sounds may be heard. In rheumatic mitral regurgitation, an opening snap (arrow) may still be heard and precedes the third heart sound (S_3) and the middiastolic murmur. Note the f wave of the apex cardiogram is co-incidental with the third heart sound (**164**).

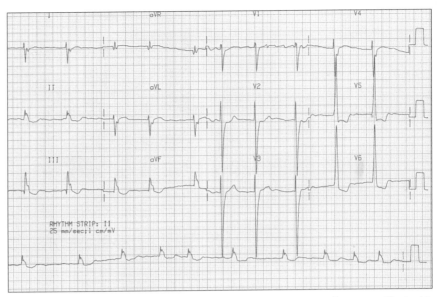

165 The electrocardiogram in non-rheumatic mitral regurgitation is usually non-specific; in this example there is atrial fibrillation and a broadened QRS with left ventricular hypertrophy, with repolarization changes (lateral and inferior ST segment depression and T wave inversion) from digoxin or ischaemia.

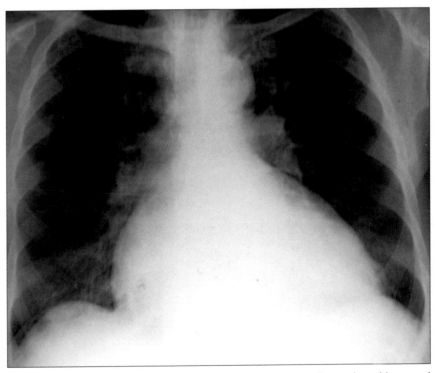

166 Chest radiograph in non-rheumatic mitral regurgitation with an enlarged heart and pulmonary congestion. The left atrium is also enlarged.

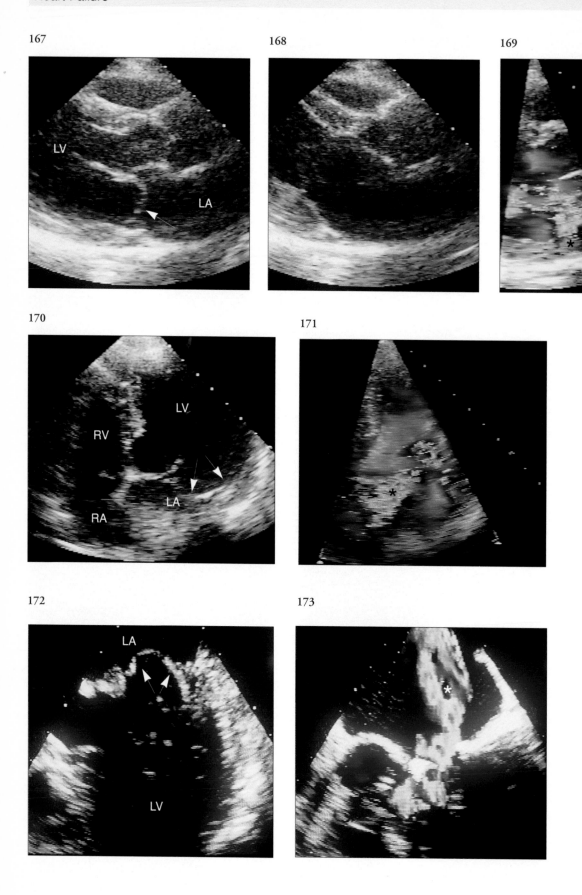

167

168

169

170

171

172

173

167–174 Echocardiograms in mitral regurgitation. Parasternal long axis view (systole, **167**; diastole, **168**), showing prolapse of the posterior mitral valve leaflet in systole (arrows) and a redundant valve with increased surface area. Colour flow Doppler demonstrates a broad regurgitant jet (*) (**169**). In an apical long axis view, the prolapsing leaflet is demonstrated (arrows) (**170**) with an eccentric and wide turbulent jet from the area of abnormal valve coaptation (*) (**171**). Transoesophageal echocardiography may be useful for assessing mitral valve prolapse (**172**) and regurgitation (by colour flow Doppler (*)) (**173**). In this case both leaflets but with particular redundancy of the posterior. Rupture of the chordae tendinae may be visualized by echocardiography and they are seen here prolapsing into the left atrium (arrow) (**174**). While mitral regurgitation may be readily detected by colour flow Doppler (**169, 171, 173**), it is not a reliable method for assessing severity.

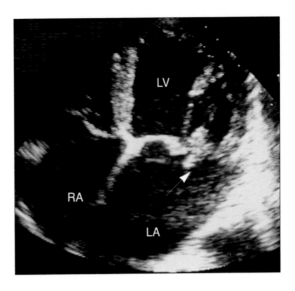

174

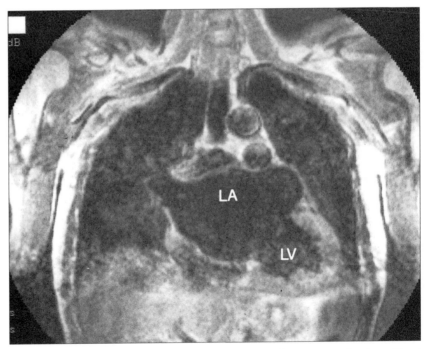

175 Magnetic resonance scan, coronal section, in severe mitral regurgitation showing a dilated left ventricle (LV) and left atrium (LA).

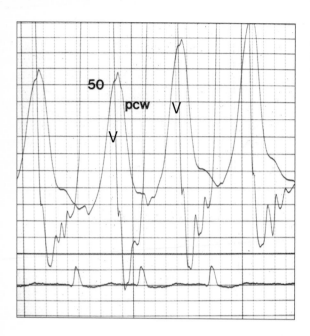

176 Haemodynamic tracing of the pulmonary capillary wedge (PCW) and left ventricular end-diastolic pressure in severe mitral regurgitation secondary to a floppy mitral valve. The *v* or systolic wave exceeds 50 mmHg. There is no gradient across the mitral valve.

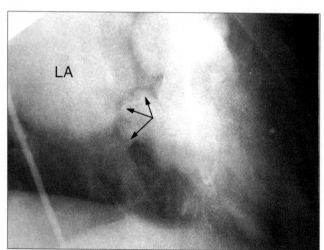

177 Left ventricular angiogram in systole showing gross mitral regurgitation through a floppy valve (arrows) as dense opacification of the left atrium (LA).

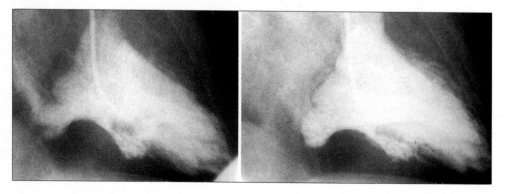

178 Left ventricular angiogram (systole left, diastole right) in mitral regurgitation with heart failure. There is severe mitral regurgitation through a localized jet in a floppy valve. The mitral annulus is considerably dilated and left ventricular function is impaired.

Chronic aortic valve disease

Aortic stenosis and regurgitation are important causes of heart failure. Aortic disease in young patients is most commonly due to a congenitally bicuspid valve which subsequently degenerates becoming stenotic or occasionally regurgitant. In older patients, degeneration of a tricuspid valve is the common form, leading to both stenosis and regurgitation. Rarer causes of aortic valve disease usually root dilatation causing regurgitation and include Marfan's syndrome, ankylosing spondylitis, Reiter's syndrome, syphilis and Ehlers–Danlos syndrome. Rheumatic heart disease may lead to aortic valve disease but is usually associated with involvement of the mitral valve.

Aortic stenosis

Obstruction to the left ventricular flow tract most commonly occurs at valvular level but may also be subvalvular or supravalvular in nature. Valvular aortic stenosis is by far the most common form in adults and children, and the non-valvular types rarely cause heart failure.

In severe aortic stenosis, cardiac output at rest is usually normal but fails to rise during exercise. Significant aortic stenosis leads to progressive concentric left ventricular hypertrophy, which is the main compensatory mechanism in the pressure-overloaded heart. However, the myocardial thickening leads to potentially adverse pathophysiological consequences. Hypertrophied myocardium has abnormal diastolic properties with disturbed filling and relaxation. Such abnormalities may lead to an increase in left atrial pressure and pulmonary venous congestion, even in the absence of reduced left ventricular contraction. When left ventricular systolic function fails, cardiac output falls and the characteristic ejection systolic murmur becomes quieter or disappears, and the slow rising arterial pulse may become more difficult to recognize. Occult aortic stenosis is an occasional cause of intractable heart failure and may be successfully treated by aortic valve replacement.

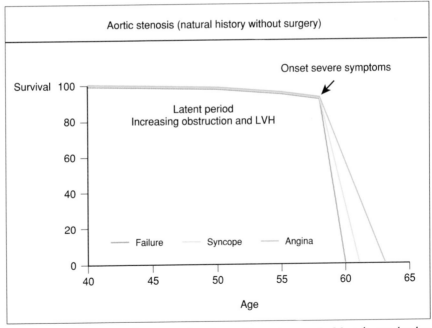

179 The natural history of unoperated patients with aortic stenosis. Most do not develop symptoms until the sixth or seventh decade. However, with the onset of severe symptoms of angina, syncope or heart failure prognosis is poor. Patients with heart failure have the worst prognosis (Ross and Braunwald, 1968).

180

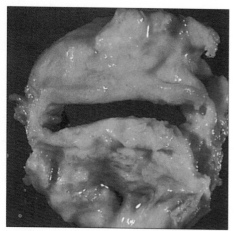

180–183 Pathology of aortic stenosis. An excised bicuspid aortic valve removed from a 72-year-old man. There was a gradient across the valve of 130 mmHg. The commissures are aligned in a left to right distribution and the cusps are heavily calcified and immobile (**180**). Rheumatic aortic stenosis occurs in a tricuspid valve with adhesions and fusion of the commissures and cusps. Calcific nodules may be present on the surface of the valve and the orifice is reduced to a triangular opening (**181**). Excised three-cuspid aortic valve which has undergone severe degeneration. Each of the three cusps is heavily calcified and immobile. The orifice is severely stenotic. Degenerative aortic valve disease is the most common cause of severe aortic stenosis in patients aged over 65 years (**182**). Transverse section through the left ventricle in aortic stenosis with ventricular hypertrophy virtually obliterating the cavity (**183**).

181

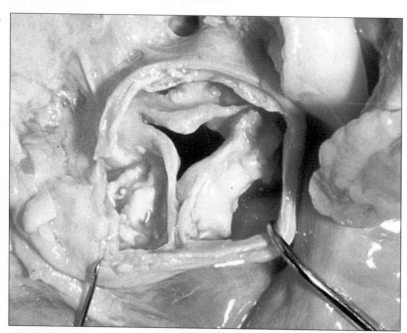

182

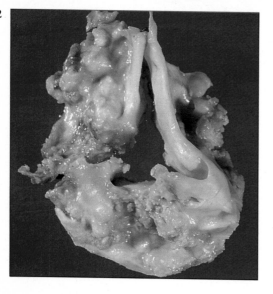

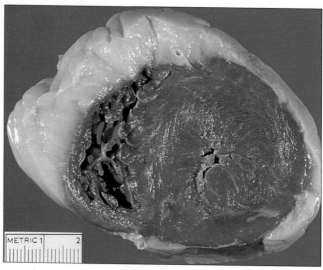

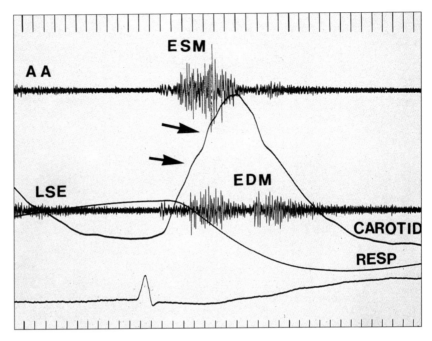

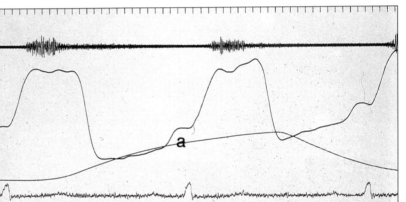

184 & 185 The physical signs on aortic stenosis are dominated by a slow rising arterial pulse, left ventricular cardiac impulse and an ejection systolic murmur. Phonocardiograms and indirect pulse recordings showing a slow rising pulse (arrow) with both an ejection systolic murmur (ESM) and an early diastolic murmur (EDM) due to mild aortic regurgitation (**184**). With increasing severity of aortic obstruction, the cardiac impulse becomes left ventricular in nature and there is a palpable *a* wave (**185**).

186

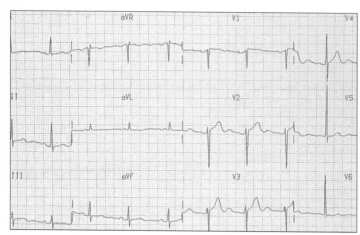

186 & 187 The electrocardiogram in aortic stenosis will show left ventricular hypertrophy with ST–T wave changes. With the onset of heart failure, left bundle branch block may be apparent as well as atrial fibrillation. In this example, left ventricular hypertrophy (deep S wave V_2, tall R waves V_{5-6}) is seen in a patient with an aortic gradient of 110 mmHg and severe breathlessness (**186**). Following surgery, the reduction in the praecordial QRS voltage is apparent (**187**).

187

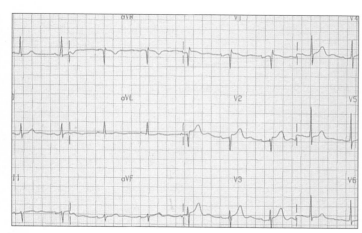

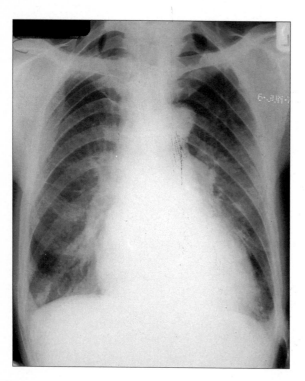

188 The chest radiograph in aortic stenosis may be normal or show left ventricular hypertrophy with a dilated ascending aorta and calcification in the aortic area. With the onset of heart failure there is cardiomegaly, upper lobe blood diversion and septal lines (Kerley B lines) indicating an increased left atrial pressure.

189–192 The echocardiogram in aortic stenosis may define the nature of the valvular abnormality and the development of left ventricular hypertrophy and impaired function. Shown here are cross-sectional views through the aortic root in a degenerative three-cusp valve with calcification and thickening along the cusp edges (**189**). The valve opens with a circular orifice (arrow). Parasternal long axis view of a calcified and immobile aortic valve with considerable left ventricular hypertrophy; systole left, diastole right (**190**). The clinical signs of heart failure may be present even in the presence of good ventricular contraction if severe hypertrophy leads to abnormal diastolic properties. Severe aortic stenosis may occur with poor ventricular function when heart failure rather than signs of aortic stenosis are the predominant feature. While left ventricular hypertrophy is still present, contraction of the left ventricle is reduced. Colour flow Doppler imaging, in a parasternal long axis echocardiographic view, shows the area of turbulent blood flow (arrow) across a calcified aortic valve (**191**). Transoesophageal echocardiography may be useful for defining the anatomy of a stenosed aortic valve; in this example, the commissures are thickened (**192**) and the orifice narrowed.

189

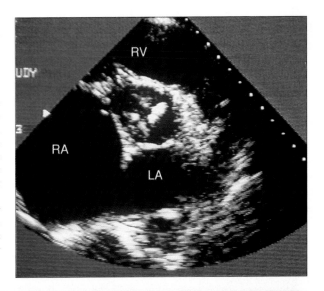

190

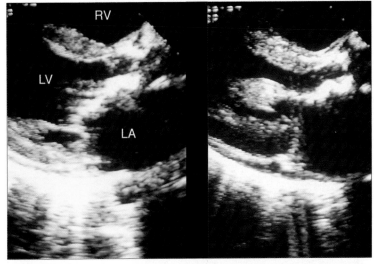

91

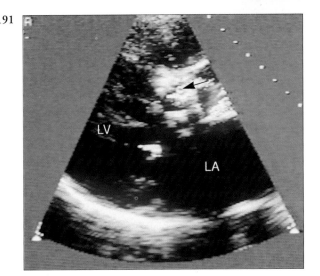

192

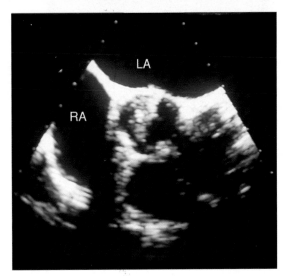

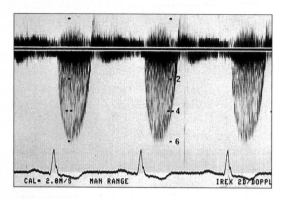

193 Continuous wave Doppler, apical view. The peak velocity of blood across the aortic valve exceeds 6 m/s suggesting the presence of severe aortic stenosis.

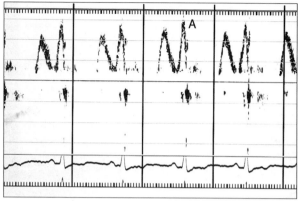

194 Pulsed wave Doppler, apical view of the mitral valve inflow, in severe aortic stenosis showing abnormal left ventricular filling. There is also a tall *a* wave (A) representing an increased contribution to left ventricular filling from atrial contraction.

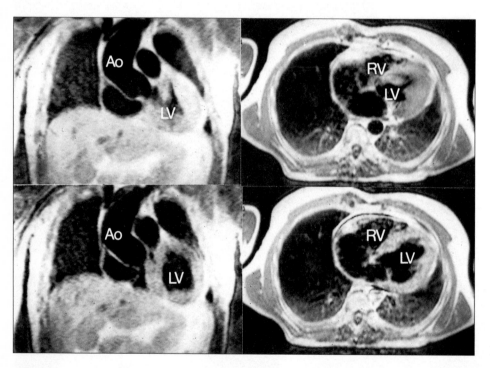

195 Magnetic resonance scans (systole above, diastole below) with coronal sections (left) and transverse section (right) in severe aortic stenosis showing marked left ventricular hypertrophy (Ao aorta, LV left ventricle, RV right ventricle).

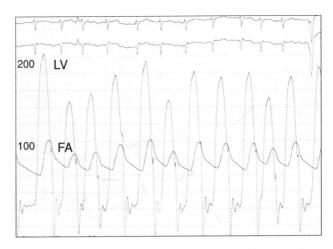

196 Haemodynamic tracing in aortic valve stenosis showing a large gradient between the left ventricular (LV) and the femoral artery (FA) in a patient with heart failure and atrial fibrillation. Note the marked beat to beat variation in the outflow gradient and the elevated end-diastolic pressure (LVEDP).

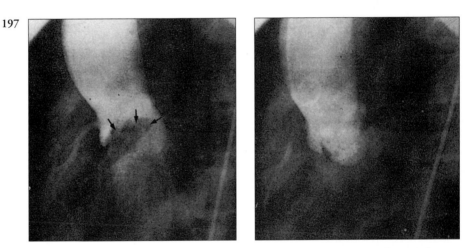

197 & 198 Aortogram in the left anterior oblique projection (systole, **197**; diastole, **198**) showing a domed stenotic aortic valve (arrows). Left ventriculography in aortic stenosis may show left ventricular hypertrophy and impaired contraction.

Subaortic and supra-aortic stenosis

Subaortic stenosis is caused by a discrete fibrous ridge, obstruction beneath the valve or by a longer fibromuscular tunnel. Supravalvular aortic stenosis is the least common form of outflow tract obstruction and is caused by localized or diffuse aortic narrowing. These forms of aortic stenosis are often associated with other heart disease and subaortic stenosis needs to be differentiated from hypertrophic cardiomyopathy. They rarely cause heart failure.

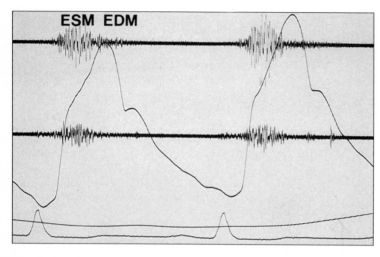

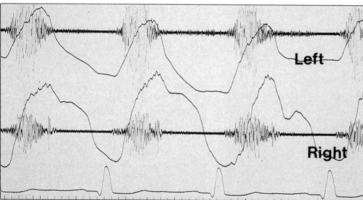

199 The physical signs in subaortic stenosis resemble hypertrophic cardiomyopathy with an ejection systolic murmur (ESM) without click, a normal second heart sound and a quiet early diastolic murmur (EDM) due to the jet interfering with aortic valve closure. The pulse is normal or brisk.

200 In supra-aortic stenosis there may be a disparity between the upstroke of the left and right carotid pulses. In this example of indirect pulse recordings, the right is slow rising and the left is slower. There is an ejection systolic murmur, loud aortic closure sound and no click.

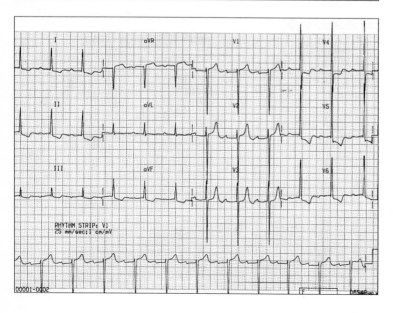

201 The electrocardiogram in these conditions will show severe left ventricular hypertrophy as in this example of supra-aortic stenosis; there is also a strain pattern and a slightly prolonged P–R interval.

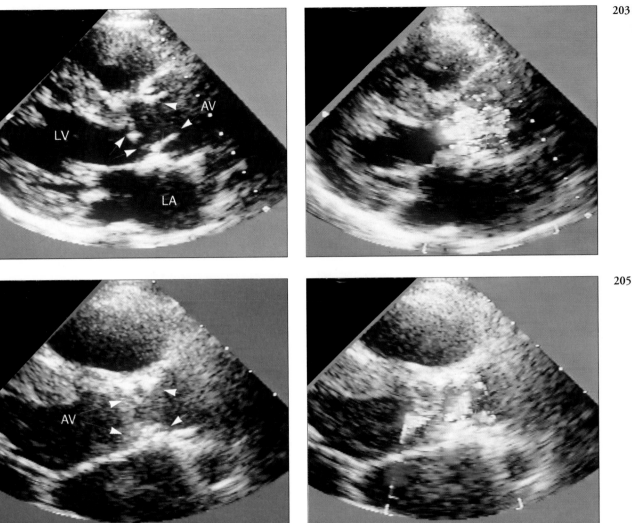

202–205 Echocardiography will define the nature of left ventricular outflow tract obstruction. In severe obstruction, left ventricular hypertrophy will be present and if heart failure has occurred systolic function may be impaired or there is other co-existing disease. Parasternal long axis view (systole, **202**) in subaortic stenosis showing a well-defined discrete membrane (arrows) below the normal looking aortic valve (AV). Colour flow Doppler defines the site of obstruction as below the aortic valve by the position of onset of turbulent blood flow (∗) (**203**). Supra-aortic stenosis often occurs with an abnormal and, in this case, thickened and stenotic aortic valve (AV). There is a diffuse area of narrowing above the valve (**204**) (arrows) which results in turbulent blood flow as seen by colour flow Doppler (**205**).

Aortic regurgitation

Patients with chronic aortic regurgitation are often symptomatic but heart failure may ensue when left ventricular function is depressed or with the onset of tachyarrhythmias. In acute aortic regurgitation, inability of the left ventricle to cope with a sudden increase in volume load leads rapidly to cardiovascular collapse and heart failure. Aortic regurgitation may be caused by abnormalities of the valve leaflets or the root or both. While rheumatic fever is the commonest form of cusp disease leading to aortic regurgitation, this is becoming less prevalent and aortic root disease is now the most commonly encountered form. In congenital bicuspid valves, aortic stenosis is the most frequent presentation though regurgitation may predominate. A number of systemic diseases are associated with aortic root dilatation such as Marfan's syndrome, Ehlers–Danlos syndrome, and ankylosing spondylitis. Many other conditions may lead to aortic root disease but are all relatively rare (**206**). Severe chronic aortic regurgitation may occur with a normal ejection fraction. There is an elevation of the left ventricular end-diastolic pressure and volume and the resultant cavity dilatation requires a rise in left ventricular systolic tension to maintain systolic pressure. These changes lead to large end-diastolic volumes with compensatory left ventricular hypertrophy. Such physiological alterations can render the patient asymptomatic for long periods. Depression of left ventricular function or worsening regurgitation usually leads to the onset of heart failure.

Causes of aortic regurgitation
Congenital valvar abnormalities (especially bicuspid valve)
Rheumatic fever
Hypertension
Marfan's syndrome
Ankylosing spondylitis
Dissection of the aorta
Familial aortic root dilatation
Infective endocarditis
Trauma
Syphilis
Aortitis
Subaortic VSD
Rheumatoid arthritis
Ehlers–Danlos syndrome
Pseudoxanthoma elasticum
Reiter's syndrome

206 Causes of aortic regurgitation.

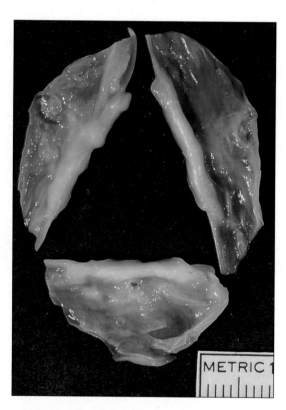

207 Excised three-cuspid valve in severe aortic regurgitation caused by disease of the aortic root. Each of the cusps is thin and delicate and mobile, similar to a normal valve. There is only slight thickening of the free edges caused by the regurgitant jet.

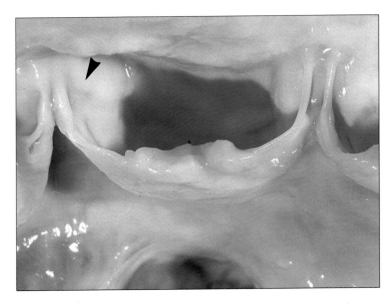

208 Aortic valve in ankylosing spondylitis with aortic regurgitation showing inflammation and thickening behind and immediately above the sinuses of Valsalva; this is particularly dense behind and adjacent to the aortic valve commissures (arrow). The valve cusps are shortened and slightly thickened.

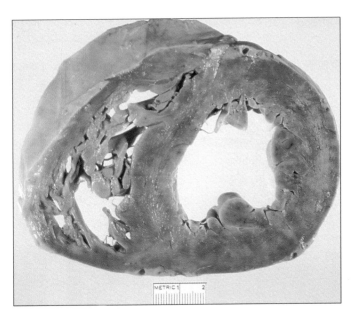

209 Transverse section through the ventricle in a patient with severe aortic regurgitation showing left ventricular cavity dilatation.

210

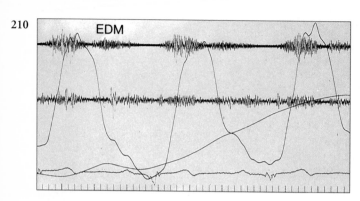

210–212 The physical signs in aortic regurgitation are dominated by a collapsing arterial pulse, displaced and heaving left ventricular impulse and an early diastolic murmur. Phonocardiograms and indirect pulse recordings in moderate aortic regurgitation. The murmur is soft and decrescendo (**210**) and best heard in expiration with the patient sitting forward (**211**). In severe aortic regurgitation, the murmur is louder and longer and may be decrescendo in form with a mid-diastolic murmur (arrows), termed an Austin Flint murmur which occurs due to vibration of the mitral valve leaflets or left ventricular wall (**212**). The indirect pulse recording shows the large volume nature of the pulse.

211

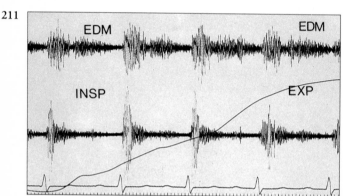

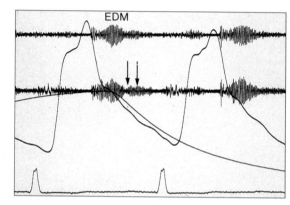

213

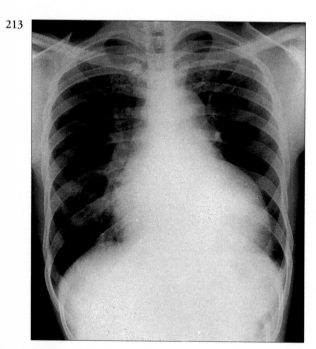

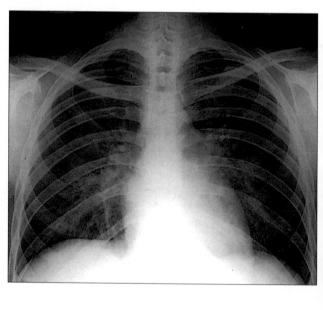

213 & 214 The investigation of aortic regurgitation in heart failure is directed towards defining its cause and severity and effect on the left ventricular function. Electrocardiography is non-specific and usually shows left ventricular hypertrophy. The chest radiograph confirms cardiomegaly and a dilated ascending aorta usually without pulmonary venous congestion (**213**). If there is acute on chronic aortic regurgitation as in infective endocarditis, there may be a rapid deterioration in ventricular function and an increase in filling pressures leading to pulmonary oedema.

215

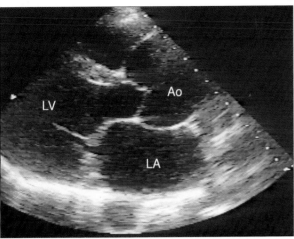

216

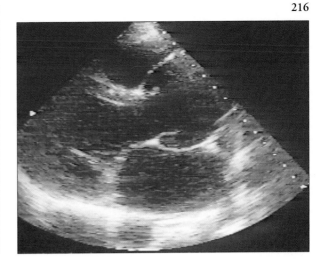

215–220 Echocardiography will usually delineate the cause of the aortic regurgitation. In aortic root disease, in this case due to Marfan's syndrome, the aortic root (Ao) becomes grossly dilated (here shown at 6 cm, normal maximum in a man 3.6 cm) leading to valvular regurgitation because of failure of leaflet coaptation and impaired left ventricular function (systole, **215**; diastole, **216**). Colour flow Doppler imaging shows a broad turbulent jet (∗) in diastole arising at the closure line of the aortic valve (**217**) and extending backwards into the left ventricle (**218**). In an apical view, the regurgitant jet is seen as a colour mosaic in early diastole extending partly (**219**) and in late diastole extending almost fully to the ventricular apex in severe aortic regurgitation (**220**).

217

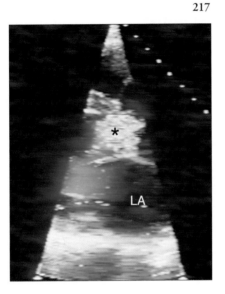

218

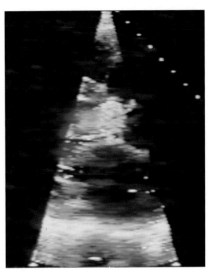

219

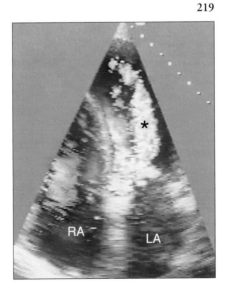

220

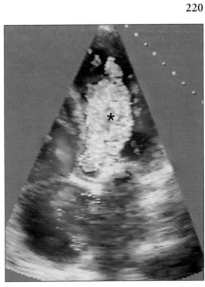

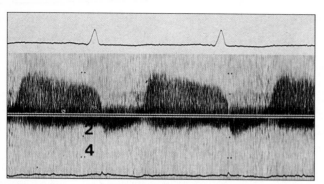

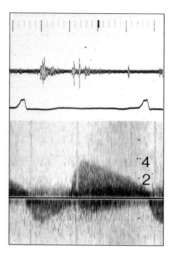

221 & 222 Aortic regurgitation may be demonstrated by Doppler ultrasound even when clinically unapparent. This may be important for patients with aortic root disease. In this example, there is a diastolic jet visualized by continuous wave Doppler from the apex (**221**). This aortic regurgitation may be defined as mild by the diastolic slope of the trace. In comparison, a similar continuous wave Doppler recording shows severe aortic regurgitation defined by a steep diastolic slope and a low aortic-left ventricular gradient at end-diastole (**222**).

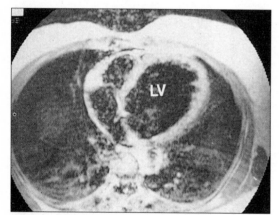

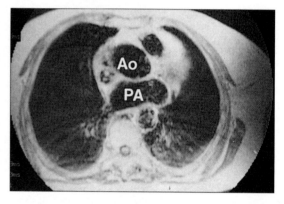

223 & 224 Magnetic resonance scans in aortic regurgitation. A dilated left ventricle (**223**), and aorta (**224**) are shown.

225 Haemodynamic tracing of a collapsing aortic pressure trace with the diastolic pressure of only 40 mmHg due to severe aortic regurgitation.

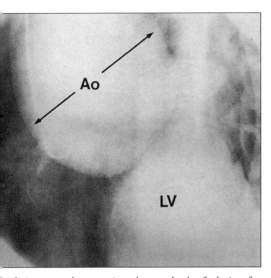

226 Aortography remains the method of choice for determining the severity of aortic regurgitation. In the left anterior oblique projection, there is a grossly dilated aortic root and ascending aorta with the left ventricle filling from free regurgitation.

Acute aortic regurgitation

Acute aortic regurgitation is usually a medical emergency, with a gravely-ill patient with tachycardia and cyanosis. There may well be pulmonary congestion and oedema. The collapsing pulse and other signs may not be as prominent as in chronic aortic regurgitation. The commonest causes of acute aortic regurgitation are aortic dissection and infective endocarditis (dealt with in a later section).

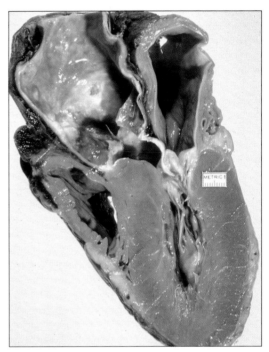

227

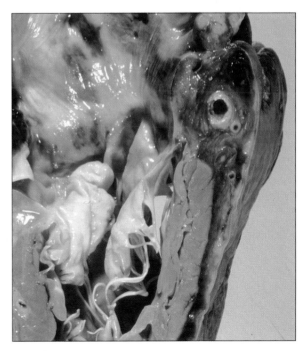

228

227 & 228 Long axis section of the heart in an 86-year-old man with aortic dissection (**227**). The descending aorta is dilated with atherosclerosis. A tear can be seen in the intima of the ascending aorta. Haemorrhage with thrombus can be seen in the false aorta channel and around the right atrioventricular sulcus to the base of the right ventricle around the coronary artery (**228**).

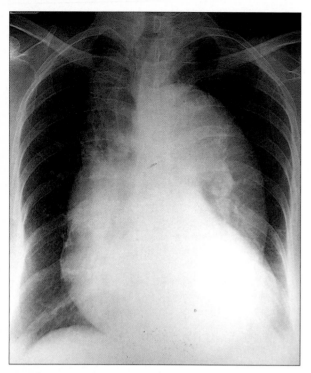

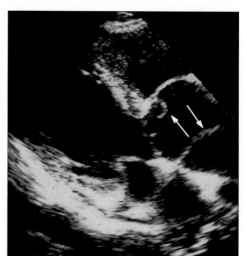

230

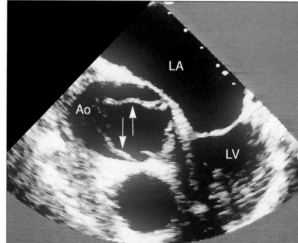

229 The chest radiograph in dissection of the aorta usually shows an enlarged, and in this case, a grossly dilated aorta. The cardiac silhouette is enlarged which may be due to ventricular dilatation or pericardial haemorrhage. In addition there is a left pleural effusion.

230–232 Transthoracic echocardiography may show the flap in aortic dissection but this is relatively unusual. An intimal flap is shown in a parasternal long axis view, both anterior and posterior, in a dilated aortic root (arrows, **230**). Transoesophageal echocardiography is now the method of choice for diagnosing aortic root dissection and a flap can be seen here in the ascending aorta (arrows) (**231**); colour flow Doppler demonstrates that the aortic valve is regurgitant (turbulent jet into the left ventricle) (∗), due to involvement by the dissection flap (**232**).

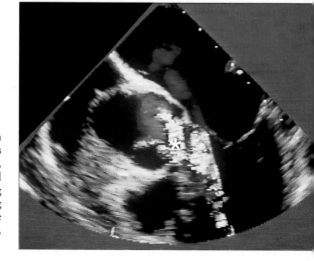

233 CT scanning will often demonstrate the presence of a dissection and the involvement of the ascending and descending aorta and, in addition, the complication of pericardial effusion. A grossly dilating ascending and descending aorta and intimal flap (arrow) is seen.

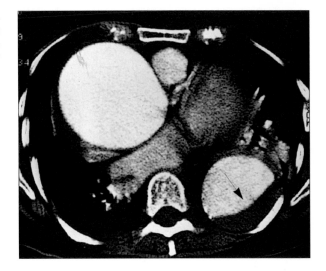

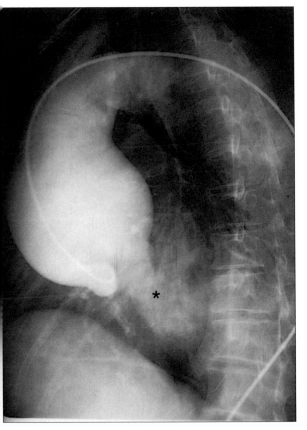

235

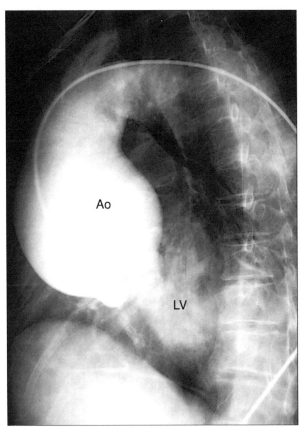

234 & 235 Aortography remains the method of choice for quantifying severity of aortic regurgitation but a dissection flap may not always be seen. Aortograph, left anterior oblique projection, shows a grossly dilated aortic root with aortic regurgitation (*) (early systole, **234**). As diastole progresses, there is a continuing leak of contrast backing to the left ventricle representing severe regurgitation (**235**).

Tricuspid valve disease

Isolated tricuspid valve disease is a very rare cause of right heart failure. Tricuspid stenosis is almost always rheumatic in origin but invariably occurs in combination with mitral valve disease. Most frequently, tricuspid regurgitation is secondary to left heart disease or pulmonary hypertension of any cause. Rarely, isolated disease of the tricuspid valve occurs due to carcinoid syndrome, Ebstein's anomaly and endocarditis especially in intravenous drug abusers. Tricuspid valve disease, particularly stenosis, is often missed clinically. The non-invasive investigation method of choice is echocardiography and Doppler. Haemodynamic investigations and angiography are often unhelpful.

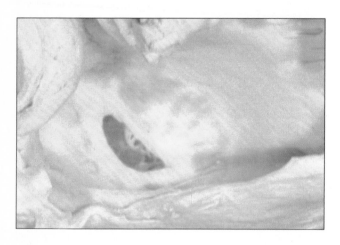

236 Stenosed tricuspid valve reviewed from above with the commissures adherent, converting the cusps into a diaphragm.

237

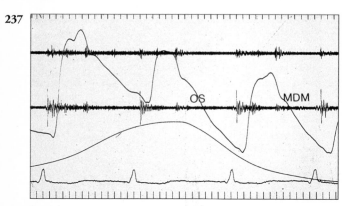

238

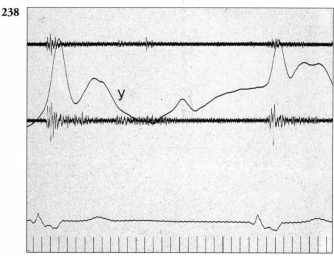

237 & 238 The physical signs of tricuspid stenosis are often difficult to detect and are masked by the co-presence of rheumatic mitral valve disease. A tricuspid opening snap and quiet mid-diastolic murmur which increases on inspiration may be heard at the right sternal edge (**237**). The characteristic abnormality is a reduced y descent in the indirectly recorded venous pressure (**238**).

239 & 240 The electrocardiogram in rheumatic mitral and tricuspid stenosis shows atrial enlargement (biphasic p wave in V1) in sinus rhythm with normal QRS morphology (**239**). Subsequently, the patient developed atrial fibrillation (**240**).

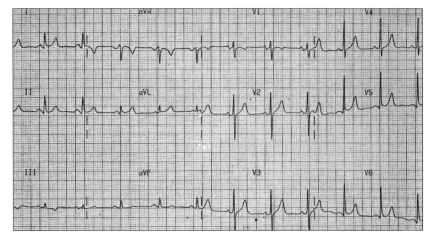

239

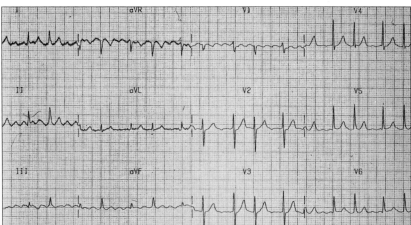

240

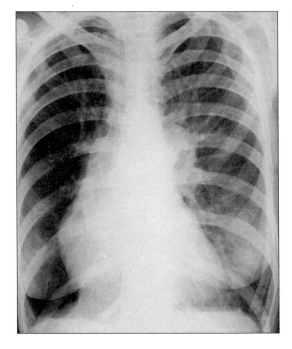

241 A chest radiograph in mixed mitral and tricuspid stenosis. There is evidence of both left and right atrial enlargement with upper lobe blood diversion.

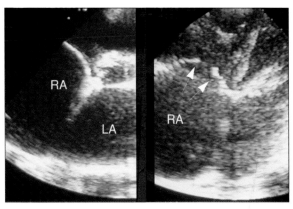

242 Echocardiogram, parasternal short axis view (left), apical long axis view (right). The stenotic tricuspid valve is thickened and domed and the right atrium enlarged (in association with mitral stenosis).

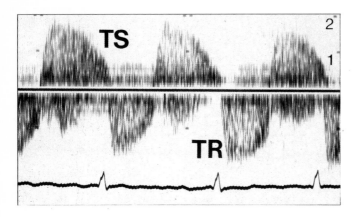

243 Tricuspid stenosis is best estimated by Doppler echocardiography. Shown here is mixed tricuspid stenosis and regurgitation.

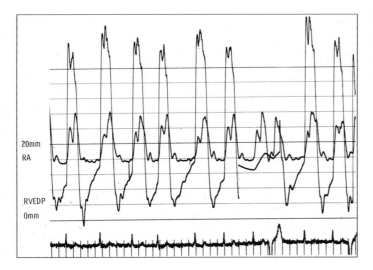

244 Haemodynamic tracing in tricuspid stenosis with a gradient across the tricuspid valve between the right atrium (RA) and right ventricular end-diastolic pressure (RVEDP). There is a tall systolic wave in the right atrial pressure trace indicating tricuspid regurgitation.

Tricuspid regurgitation

Tricuspid regurgitation is most commonly due not to an intrinsic abnormality of the valve itself, but to dilatation of the right ventricle and tricuspid annulus. This may be a complication of right ventricular failure or pulmonary hypertension of any cause. Very rarely, it may be due to an anatomically abnormal valve such as may occur in rheumatic heart disease, infective endocarditis, Ebstein's anomaly, floppy valve or carcinoid syndrome. Infective endocarditis is dealt with in a later section.

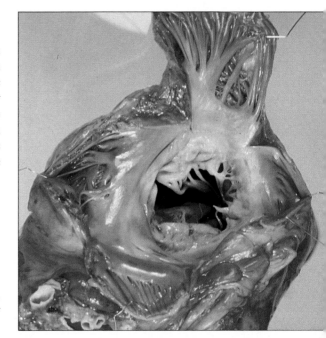

245 The tricuspid valve seen through the open right atrium. There is dilatation of the tricuspid ring due to pulmonary hypertension secondary to left heart disease.

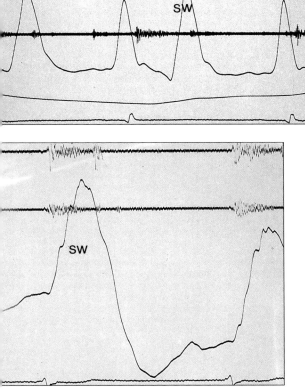

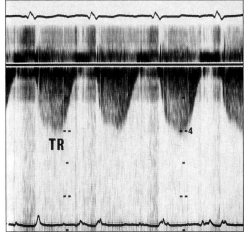

248

249

250

246 & 247 The physical signs in tricuspid regurgitation are dominated by the presence of a systolic wave in the venous pressure. There may be a pansystolic murmur but this is often quiet. When a patient is in sinus rhythm, there will be an accentuated *a* wave (a) as well as a systolic wave (SW) here shown on indirect recordings (**246**). With the onset of atrial fibrillation, the *a* wave will be absent and only a systolic wave is observed (**247**).

248–250 Tricuspid regurgitation may be found by echocardiography in some normal individuals. Echocardiography may reveal the aetiology of the regurgitation but it is often unhelpful in assessing severity. The most common finding is a dilated tricuspid annulus with failure of coaptation of the leaflets. In these examples of pulmonary hypertension with secondary tricuspid regurgitation, a normal (**248**) and an enlarged right ventricle and right atrium (**249**) are seen. There is a broad and turbulent jet of tricuspid regurgitation extending into the right atrium. Continuous wave Doppler may be useful for documenting the presence of tricuspid regurgitation and, more importantly, the severity of pulmonary hypertension. In this example (**250**), the regurgitant jet is 4 m/s which equates to a right ventricular pressure of approximately 64 mmHg.

Carcinoid syndrome

Tricuspid regurgitation is a common manifestation of carcinoid syndrome. This occurs due to focal or diffuse deposits of fibrous tissue on the endocardium of the valve cusps. White fibrous carcinoid plaques are extensively deposited on the right side of the heart. They most often lead to tricuspid regurgitation, although tricuspid stenosis and pulmonary valve disease may also occur as well as, much less frequently, left-sided valvular lesions.

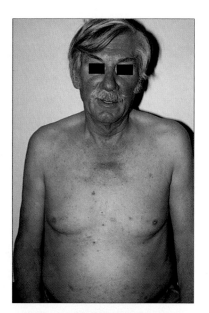

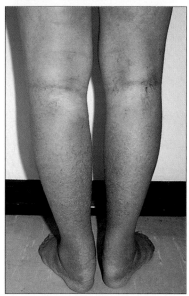

252 & 253 A patient with carcinoid syndrome will initially have flushing episodes which may lead on to persistent peripheral and facial vasodilatation as seen here in the face and abdomen (**252**, top) and legs (**253**, bottom).

Site of origin of carcinoid tumours

Appendix

Rectum

Bowel (other)

Ovary
Pancreas
Stomach
Caecum

Ileum

Lung

251 Frequency distribution of the site of origin of carcinoid tumours. The biochemical effect of these tumours is not apparent until there has been metastasis to the liver. The vasomotor, bronchoconstrictor and cardiac manifestations are related to circulating humoral substances secreted by the tumour (National Cancer Institute, 1950–71).

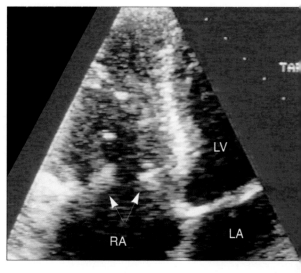

254 The echocardiogram of the tricuspid valve has a characteristic appearance as the valve is thickened in a half-opened, half-closed position (arrows). This predominantly leads to tricuspid regurgitation though the valve may also be stenotic.

Heart failure following cardiac surgery

Heart failure may become apparent immediately following, or some time after, cardiac surgery. Valve dysfunction, impaired left ventricular function and arrhythmias may, singly or in combination, be responsible. Perioperative myocardial infarction or poor pre-operative left ventricular function may result in immediate or delayed heart failure. Prosthetic valves may develop dehiscence of the sewing ring resulting in severe paravalvular regurgitation especially related to endocarditis. Inadequate anticoagulation, especially in metallic valves, may lead to thrombotic obstruction and stenosis. Bioprostheses may degenerate and become stenotic or regurgitant, such changes occurring rapidly in the presence of infection. Conservative mitral surgery may rarely be followed by acute severe regurgitation. Such changes may lead to the rapidly progressive or insidious onset of dyspnoea or heart failure. Investigation is directed towards detection of the valvular dysfunction and assessing left ventricular contraction.

Mitral valve surgery

Mitral valve surgery includes valvotomy which may be open or closed in approach, or mitral valve repair or replacement.

255 Physical signs in a patient with mitral re-stenosis: there is an opening snap (OS) and a mid-diastolic murmur. Re-stenosis may occur early or late following surgery but is less common following open valvotomy undertaken on cardiopulmonary bypass.

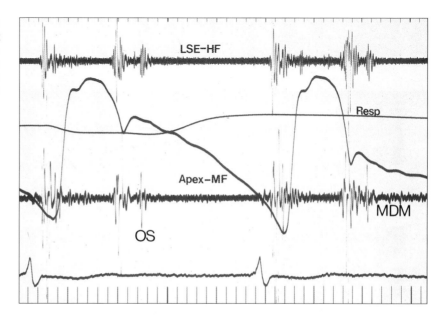

256 & 257 Chest radiographs in a patient following mitral valvotomy (**256**). Nine years later, pulmonary oedema occurred due to valvular re-stenosis (**257**).

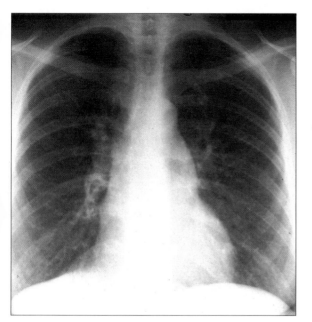

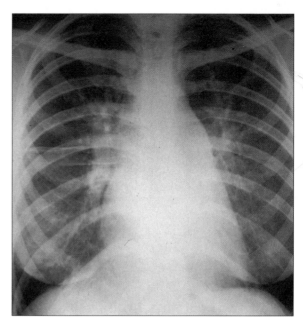

257

258

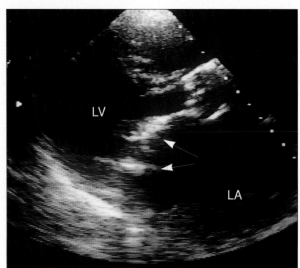

258 Echocardiogram, parasternal long axis view, showing re-stenosis of the mitral valve (arrows). Imaging of the valve to measure the orifice area is not reliable following valvotomy and the Doppler pressure half-time method should be used.

259

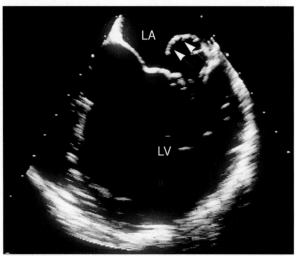

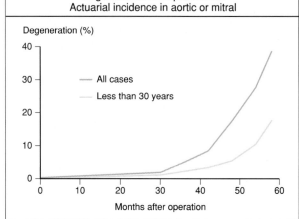

259 & 260 Following mitral valve repair, there is usually a prolonged period with no or only minimal regurgitation. Heart failure may occur if severe mitral regurgitation develops or left ventricular function deteriorates. Echocardiogram, trans-oesophageal four chamber view, showing prolapse of both mitral valve leaflets with ruptured chordae (arrows) (**259**). Following repair with an annular ring (arrows) and quadrantic resection, and despite the lack of regurgitation, the patient developed heart failure due to poor left ventricular function (**260**).

261 The degeneration of biological valve prostheses may be assessed on an actuarial basis. After five years, 40 per cent of patients over the age of 30 will have sustained a degree of valve failure (Williams *et al.*, 1980).

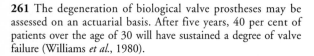

262 An excised mitral xenograft which is calcified and degenerative.

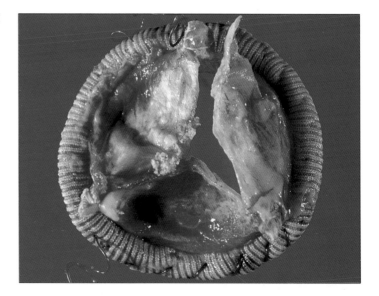

263 Echocardiogram, parasternal long axis view, systole left, diastole right. A xenograft mitral valve is seen which prolapses into the left atrium in systole (arrow) leading to severe regurgitation.

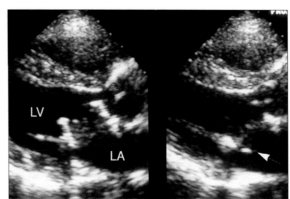

265

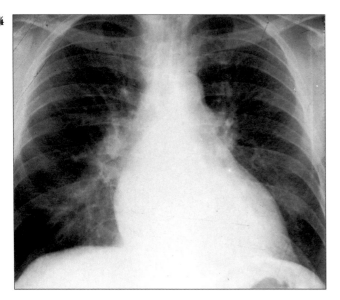

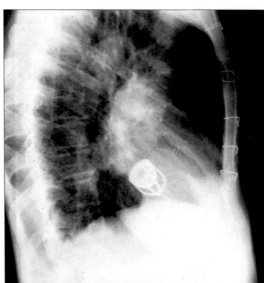

264 & 265 Chest radiographs (posteroanterior, **264**; lateral, **265**) showing pulmonary oedema secondary to a paraprosthetic leak following a Starr–Edwards mitral valve replacement.

266

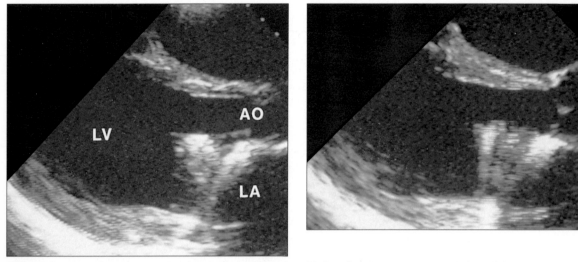

266 & 267 Echocardiograms, parasternal long axis view (systole, **266**; diastole, **267**), in a patient with heart failure due to poor left ventricular function in the presence of a normally functioning Starr–Edwards mitral valve replacement.

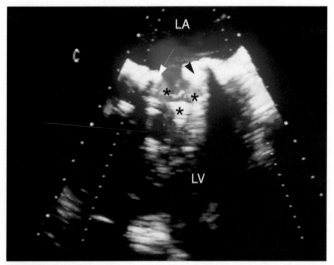

268 Transoesophageal echocardiography may be useful to examine the function of prosthetic valves. In this example, there is a normally functioning Björk–Shiley mitral valve (sewing ring marked by arrows) without left atrial thrombus. There is little detail seen of the valve because of interference (∗) to the ultrasound by the prosthetic valve material.

Aortic valve surgery

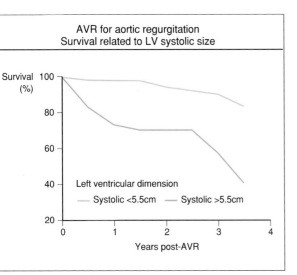

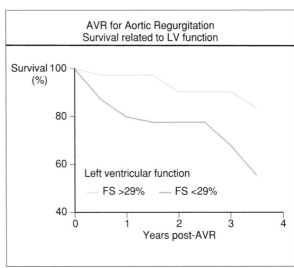

269 & 270 Following aortic valve surgery for stenosis, even if the preoperative left ventricular contraction is poor and heart failure is present, a good long-term outcome can be achieved. However, in aortic regurgitation, if there is preoperative left ventricular dilatation (systolic dimension **269**, Bonow *et al., 1980*) or poor contraction (**270**, Bonow *et al.*, 1982), survival is impaired and heart failure occurs much more frequently.

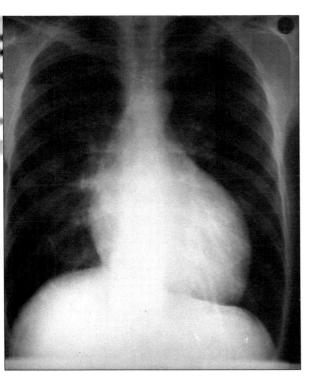

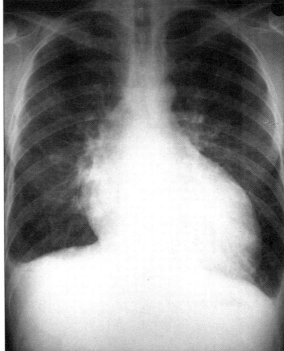

271 & 272 Chest radiograph immediately following an aortic valve replacement for aortic regurgitation (**271**). The valve was initially competent but heart failure ensued when the paravalvular regurgitation occurred (**272**).

273 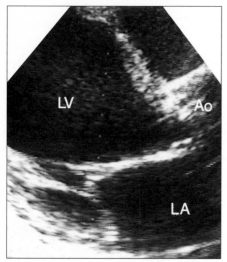 274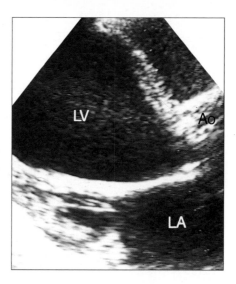

273 & 274 Echocardiograms (systole, **273**; diastole, **274**) in a patient who had a competent aortic valve replacement but who suffered heart failure due to poor left ventricular function.

4. HEART MUSCLE DISEASE

Heart failure may result from myocardial disease: this may be due to underlying ischaemic, hypertensive, congenital or valvular causes. These conditions may be of unknown aetiology and classified as cardiomyopathies (dilated, hypertrophic or restrictive) or as due to known causes and therefore defined as specific heart muscle disorders. The origins of myocardial disease are varied and include inflammatory, metabolic, endocrine, nutritional, toxic, infiltrative, fibroplastic, haematological, genetic, and post-partum causes (**275**).

Cardiomyopathies and specific heart muscle disorders may lead to heart failure by impairment of systolic ventricular contraction, abnormal diastolic properties of the left ventricle, restriction in ventricular filling or secondary valvular abnormalities. Diagnosis of such disorders is by the identification of specific features and endomyocardial biopsy or by a process of exclusion. By far the most common disorders are dilated and hypertrophic cardio-myopathies. The remainder of the heart muscle diseases are rare in western countries although in other parts of the world some are relatively common.

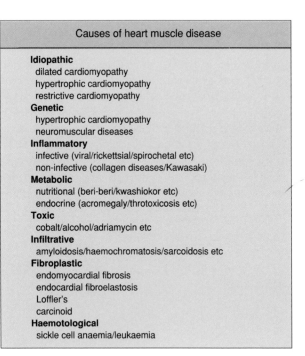

275 Causes of heart muscle disease.

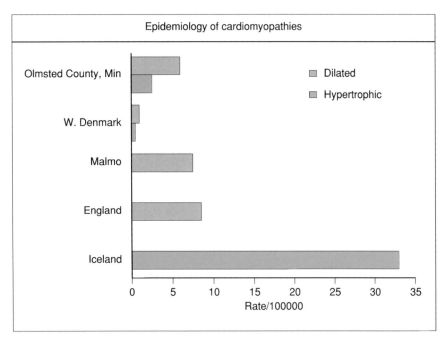

276 The relative distribution of hypertrophic and dilated cardiomyopathies in a number of Western countries. There appears to be a large variation in the incidence of these disorders; whether this is real is unclear (Codd *et al.*, 1989).

Idiopathic dilated cardiomyopathy

Idiopathic dilated cardiomyopathy is defined as a 'dilated left ventricle with poor contraction'. This disorder is probably of multifactorial origin and is the final common pathway for a number of causes of myocardial damage produced by toxic, metabolic or infectious agents. It is probable that, at least in some cases, the cause is viral myocarditis but this has not been finally established. At post-mortem there may be enlargement of all four cardiac chambers and particularly of the left ventricle. Ventricular hypertrophy is minimal and on microscopy extensive areas of interstitial and perivascular fibrosis are seen.

The symptoms in idiopathic dilated cardiomyopathy may be of insidious onset. Patients may remain asymptomatic with left ventricular dilatation for a considerable period. The clinical course, however, is usually one of progressive deterioration with three-quarters of the patients dying within the first five years of the onset of symptoms. Less frequently, severe heart failure develops acutely during an attack of apparent myocarditis. Physical examination is non-specific showing low cardiac output, congestive heart failure and cardiac enlargement. Echocardiography shows dilatation of the left ventricle, and coronary angiography and myocardial biopsy may be required to exclude other causes of heart muscle disease. Other secondary causes include alcoholism, rheumatic fever, myoedema, acromegaly, storage disorders, sarcoidosis, phaeochromocytoma, renal failure, neuromuscular conditions, adriamycin toxicity and scleroderma. Rarely, dilated cardiomyopathy may occur in pregnancy.

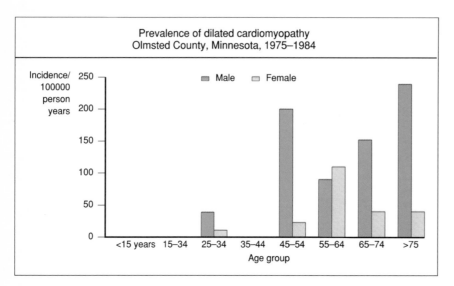

277 The age and sex distribution of cases of dilated cardiomyopathy in Olmsted County, Minnesota, from 1975–84. This disease is predominantly found in middle-aged men and is less frequent in women (Codd *et al.*, 1989).

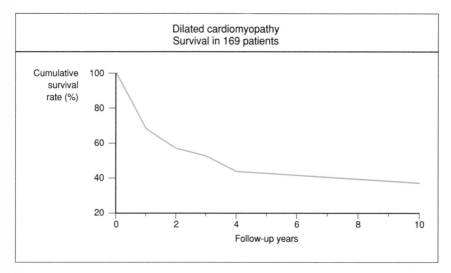

278 Dilated cardiomyopathy has an extremely poor prognosis. Less than 50 per cent of patients survive five years (Diaz *et al.*, 1987).

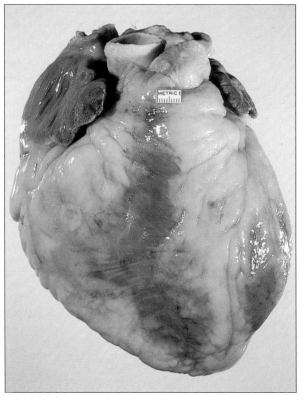
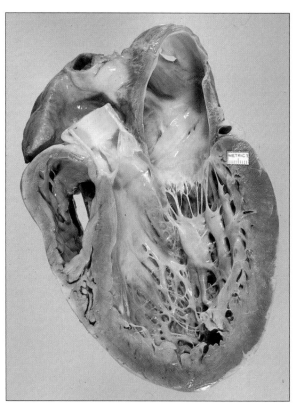

279 & 280 Macroscopic view of the heart in dilated cardiomyopathy. The heart is enlarged and there may be a considerable increase in heart weight (**279**). The long axis echocardiographic cut showed a grossly dilated left ventricular cavity. The myocardium is not hypertrophied and there are white areas of fibrosis overlying the endocardium, which are related to local thrombosis secondary to blood stasis (**280**).

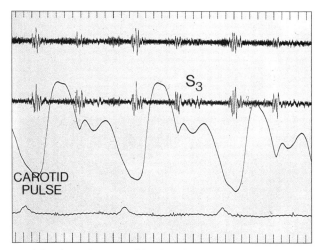

281 The physical signs in dilated cardiomyopathy are non-specific showing a small volume arterial pulse, third and fourth heart sounds with a summation gallop, elevated venous pressure and secondary tricuspid regurgitation. In this example, a small volume carotid pulse (indirect recording) and third heart sound are seen.

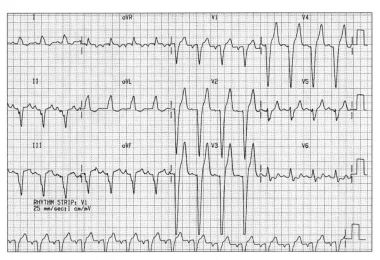

282 The electrocardiogram in idiopathic dilated cardiomyopathy is non-specific and may show anterior praecordial Q waves or alternatively, as in this case, left bundle branch block. Atrial enlargement is frequently seen, with atrial fibrillation being a common complication; this can lead to clinical deterioration and embolism. Ventricular tachyarrhythmias are also frequently observed and may be the cause of sudden death.

283
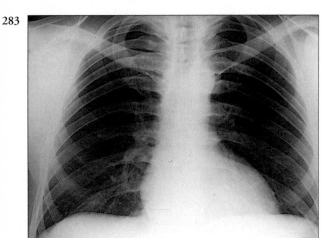
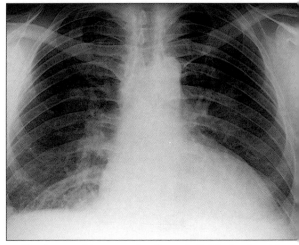

283 & 284 The chest radiograph in dilated cardiomyopathy is non-specific. A man with a normal radiograph (**283**), developed heart failure and cardiomegaly two years later; pulmonary venous congestion became apparent (**284**).

285
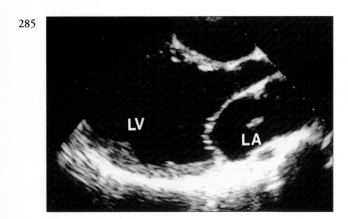
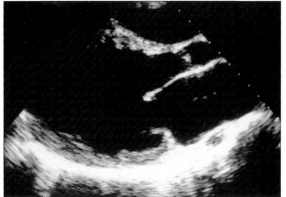

287

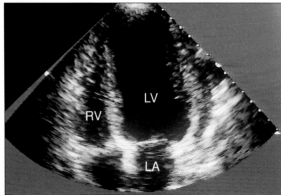

288

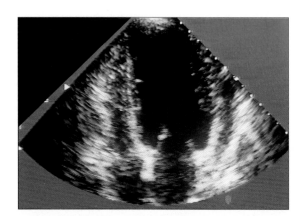

289

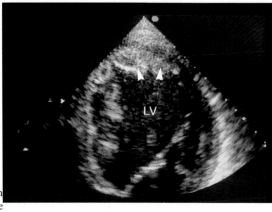

285–290 Echocardiography in dilated cardiomyopathy reveals a dilated, poorly functioning left ventricle as the primary abnormality. The right ventricle and both atria may be dilated, and a pericardial effusion or mural thrombus may be present. Colour flow Doppler frequently demonstrates the presence of mitral and tricuspid regurgitation. A long axis parasternal view in dilated cardiomyopathy (systole, **285**; diastole, **286**) showing a dilated left ventricle which contracts very poorly. There is no compensatory left ventricular hypertrophy. The apical view gives further information about global left ventricular contraction. In this example, there is generalized poor function (systole, **287**; diastole, **288**). The development of atrial and ventricular intracavity thrombus (arrows) is a major complication of cardiomyopathy and may lead to systolic embolization (**289**). Colour flow Doppler imaging shows a jet of mitral regurgitation due to dilatation of the mitral annulus and papillary muscle malalignment; usually this is not severe. A jet of mitral regurgitation into a large left atrium may be seen. Continuous wave Doppler frequently shows the presence of mitral regurgitation. In this case (**290**), there is a slow upstroke of the regurgitant jet (arrow) representing a reduced rate of rise of ventricular pressure, due to poor contraction.

290

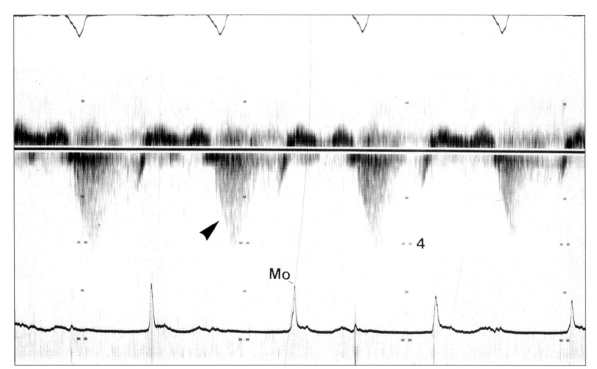

291

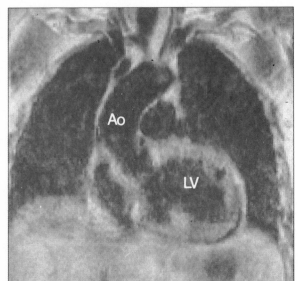

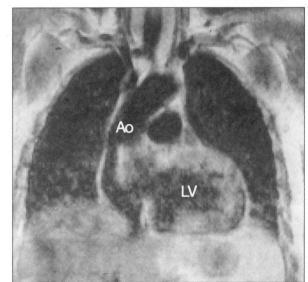

293

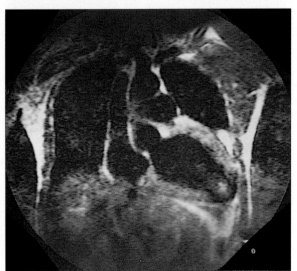

291–293 Magnetic resonance scanning may define ventricular cavity size and contraction, myocardial hypertrophy and the presence of intracavity thrombus. In this example, there is a dilated poorly contracting left ventricle with some compensatory hypertrophy. There is a small pericardial effusion sited at the apex (systole, **291**; diastole, **292**). In a sagittal section there is a large apical thrombus (**293**).

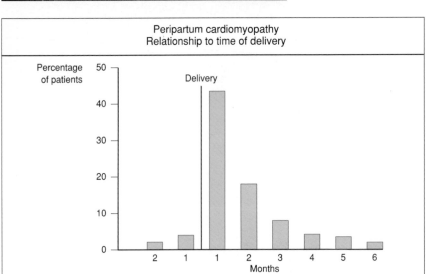

294 Peripartum cardiomyopathy is a condition indistinguishable from idiopathic dilated cardiomyopathy which occurs around the time of delivery; spontaneous recovery may occur but the condition may recur with subsequent pregnancies (Homans, 1985).

Myocarditis

A number of inflammatory processes due to infectious agents may involve the heart. Myocarditis may be caused by a variety of viral, rickettsial, bacterial, protozoal and metazoal diseases. Myocarditis can be an acute or chronic process and in western countries viruses are by far the most common agents of the disease. Clinical cases of myocarditis may vary from an unrecognized and self-limiting episode to a life-threatening illness presenting as acute heart failure or arrhythmia.

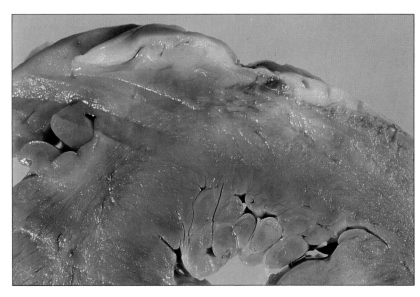

295

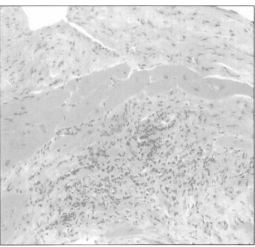

296

295 & 296 Myocarditis may be seen pathologically with a wide variety of changes. The heart may be dilated, hypertrophied or flabby and there may be inflammatory reaction with myocytolysis and necrosis. In this example (**295**), in a young man who died with acute myocarditis, the left ventricular wall is mottled with focal pale areas which are mainly subepicardial, having some patches of darker discoloration which are neurotic. Left ventricular biopsy specimen in acute viral myocarditis (**296**). There is fibrosis of the myocardium (top) with a lymphocytic infiltrate (below).

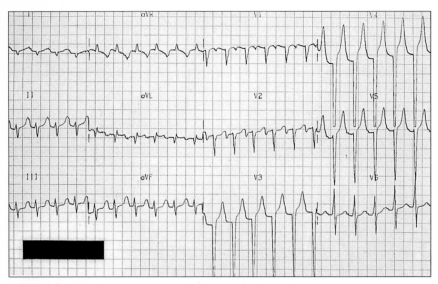

297 The electrocardiogram in myocarditis is non-specific. In this example, there is left atrial enlargement with left bundle branch block. The pattern of myocardial infarction is quite commonly seen and may lead to diagnostic difficulties.

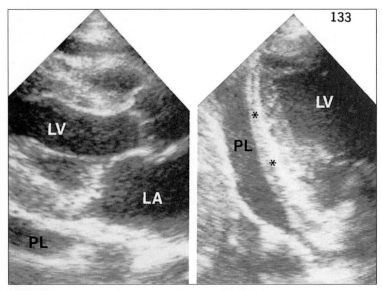

298 Echocardiogram, parasternal long axis view (left), apical long axis view (right), in myopericarditis: pericardial (∗) and pleural (PL) effusions are common. The pericardium is grossly thickened and there is impairment of ventricular contraction.

Hypertrophic cardiomyopathy

Hypertrophic cardiomyopathy is defined as 'idiopathic hypertrophy of a non-dilated left ventricle'. It is usually transmitted as an autosomal dominant trait, although non-familial cases occur. The distribution of left ventricular hypertrophy is characteristically asymmetrical septal but may occur symmetrically or at the apex. The hypertrophied left ventricle frequently demonstrates abnormal diastolic properties including impaired relaxation and filling. This leads to an elevated left ventricular filling and left atrial pressure. Therefore, despite a hypercontractive left ventricle, patients may present with breathlessness and heart failure. While ventricular tachyarrhythmias are a cause of syncope and death, atrial tachyarrhythmias, particularly atrial fibrillation, may lead to the onset of heart failure.

299 Incidence of hypertrophic cardiomyopathy in Olmsted County, Minnesota, 1975–84. The disease appears to be more common in younger men and older women; however, it may present in any age from infancy to the sixth or seventh decade (Codd *et al.*, 1989).

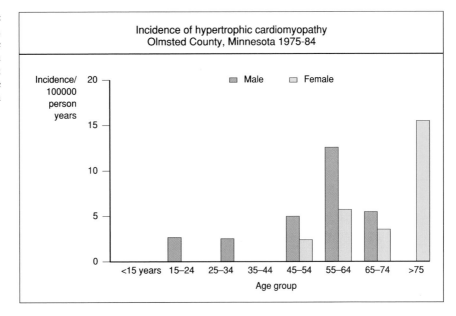

300 The cause of death in hypertrophic cardiomyopathy is sudden or unexpected in more than half the cases due to ventricular arrhythmias, and in a third of cases due to cardiac failure (Mckenna, 1988).

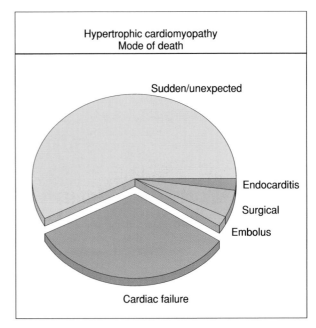

301

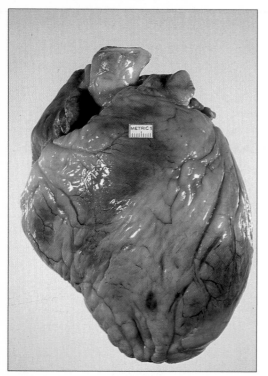

302

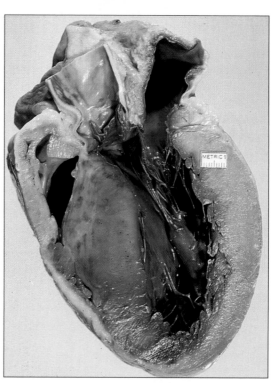

301 & 302 The external appearance of the heart in hypertrophic cardiomyopathy. There is a marked increase in cardiac weight due to left ventricular hypertrophy (**301**). In the long axis echo cut (**302**), there is gross left ventricular hypertrophy, more marked in the septum than in the free wall.

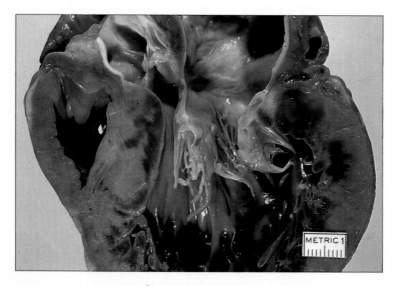

303 Long axis section of the heart in non-obstructive hypertrophic cardiomyopathy. The mitral valve is abnormal with severe thickening of both leaflets and some chordae which give the valve a 'cartilaginous' consistency. This appearance of the mitral valve is common in patients with hypertrophic cardiomyopathy and results from abnormal leaflet coaptation. The development of mitral regurgitation in hypertrophic cardiomyopathy is often associated with left atrial enlargement and supraventricular arrhythmias as well as the development of heart failure.

304 Excised septal myocardium from a patient with hypertrophic obstructive cardiomyopathy who underwent a myotomy and myectomy. The thickened white endocardium occurs at the point of contact between the septum and mitral valve during systole. Surgical removal of part of the thickened ventricular septum is effective in reducing the left ventricular outflow tract gradient. In selected patients, it may be the treatment of choice for the relief of angina or heart failure.

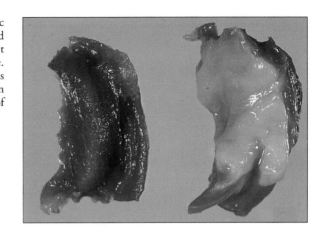

305 & 306 Histological sections of the ventricular septum in hypertrophic cardiomyopathy. A high-powered view shows thickened intramural coronary arteries, especially of the media and the intima. There is considerable luminal narrowing. Adjacent to the thickened arteries, are areas of fibrosis in the myocardium (**305**). There is marked fibre disarray (**306**) and there are areas of fibrosis between fibres; the hypertrophied fibres are malaligned with larger nuclei.

305

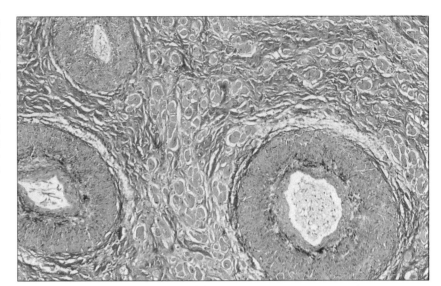

306
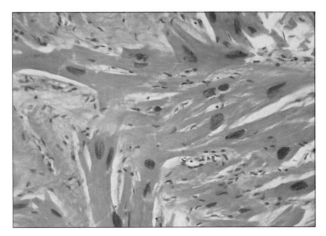

307

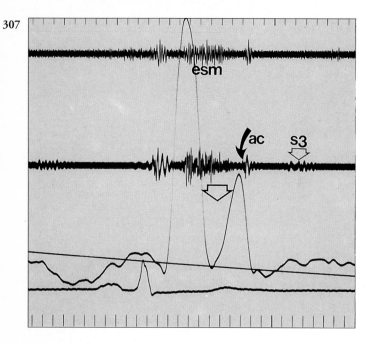

esm

ac s3

307–310 Physical examination of hypertrophic cardiomyopathy reveals an ejection systolic murmur and delay in aortic valve closure (black arrow). A third heart sound (s_3) and/or a fourth heart sound may be present (**307**). The carotid pulse (indirect recording) is jerky due to mid-systolic left ventricular outflow obstruction causing collapse of the pulse (broad arrow). Characteristically, the ejection systolic murmur in hypertrophic cardiomyopathy is accentuated by the Valsalva manoeuvre and post-extrasystolic potentiation. A ventricular extrasystole (VE) causes an increase in the ejection systolic murmur in a post-extrasystolic beat (**308**). The cardiac impulse becomes sustained representing left ventricular hypertrophy with a tall *a* wave (a) and there may be a palpable fourth heart sound (S_4) (**309**). In patients without heart failure, the jugular venous pressure may be elevated due to the Bernheim effect which stimulates right ventricular hypertrophy and pulmonary stenosis due to bulging of the ventricular septum into the right ventricle. The venous pressure therefore shows a tall *a* wave (**310**). With the onset of heart failure, cardiac enlargement and increasing mitral regurgitation may result in the loss of outflow tract gradient.

308

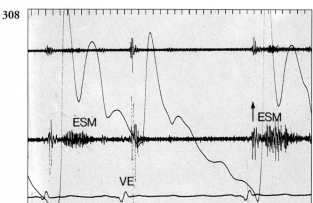

ESM

ESM

VE

309

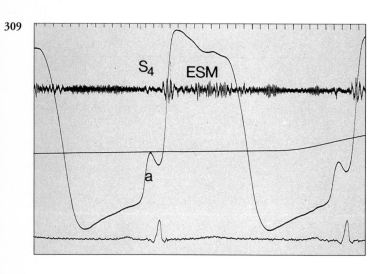

S_4 ESM

a

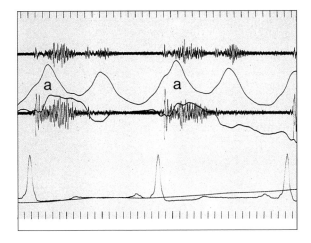

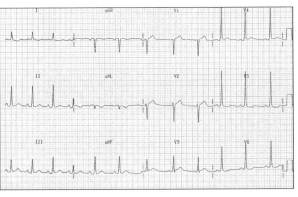

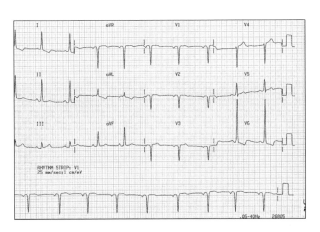

311–313 The electrocardiogram in hypertrophic cardiomyopathy is variable but usually shows severe left ventricular hypertrophy with lateral ST segment depression. Left atrial enlargement and pathological Q waves are common in hypertrophied cardiomyopathy, even in the absence of clinical or pathological evidence of myocardial infarction. They probably represent extensive myocardial fibrosis and are not uncommon in patients with heart failure. In this series, the initial ECG shows atrial and left ventricular hypertrophy (**311**). Two years later, with the onset of severe dyspnoea, there is loss of praecordial R waves, ST segment depression and T wave inversion in V6, I and AVL (**312**). Following resection of an outflow tract obstruction, left bundle branch block is evident: the rhythm is atrial flutter with 2:1 conduction post-operatively (**313**).

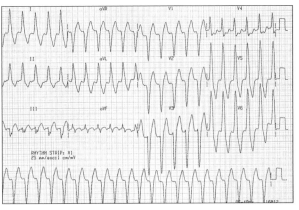

314 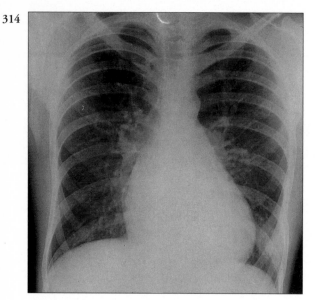 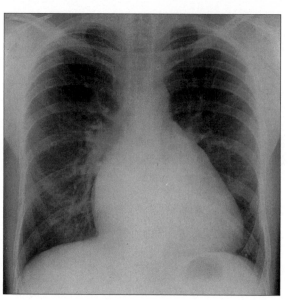 315

314 & 315 The chest radiograph in hypertrophic cardiomyopathy may be normal (**314**). Three years later, (**315**) the heart is enlarged with upper lobe blood diversion.

316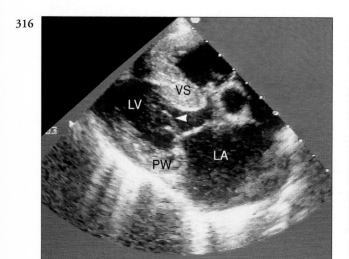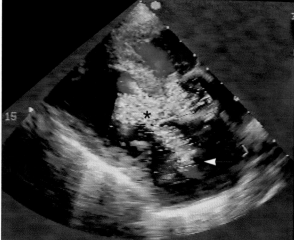

316–320 Echocardiography is an investigation of choice for the diagnosis of hypertrophic cardiomyopathy. There is moderate hypertrophy of the interventricular septum (VS) with a small left ventricular cavity and systolic anterior motion of the mitral valve (arrow) (**316**). Colour flow Doppler shows the outflow tract obstruction to be at the site of mitral–septal apposition (∗) and the coexisting mitral regurgitation is seen as a turbulent mosaic jet (arrow) (**317**). Hypertrophy, particularly in younger age groups, may be symmetrical with equal thickening of the septum and posterior wall which can be seen in a parasternal long axis view (**318**) but better appreciated on a parasternal short axis view with the septum (VS) and posterior wall (PW) of equal thickness. The left ventricular cavity is reduced in size (**319**). Transoesophageal echocardiography may be useful for defining the extent and severity of left ventricular hypertrophy and the presence of a left ventricular outflow tract obstruction in patients in whom transthoracic echocardiography produces unsatisfactory images. In this example, there is marked ventricular septal hypertrophy (**320**).

318

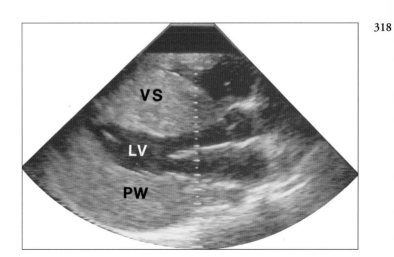

319

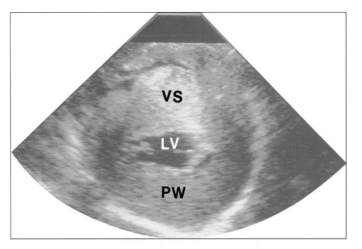

320

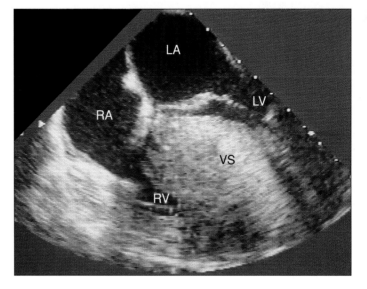

321

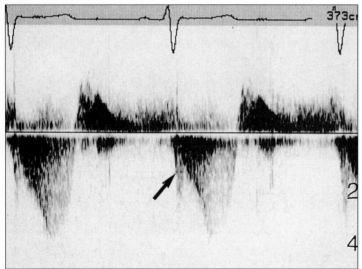

321 & 322 Doppler echocardiography (continuous wave from the apex) demonstrates the severity of outflow tract gradient; initially in systole there is trivial mitral regurgitation (arrow) and then a slow rising mid-systolic gradient from the left ventricular outflow obstruction (**321**). Pulsed Doppler of the mitral inflow may demonstrate the abnormal filling and relaxation properties of the left ventricle in hypertrophic cardiomyopathy. In this example (**322**), taken from the apex, there is reduced rate of initial flow (arrow) and a tall *a* wave suggesting an increased atrial contribution to left ventricular filling (**322**).

322

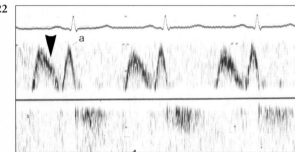

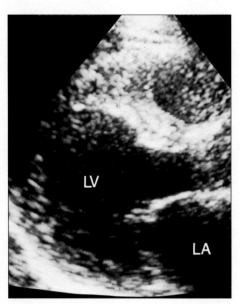

323 Heart failure usually occurs in patients with hyperdynamic left ventricular function. Occasionally, dilatation of the ventricle occurs due to myocardial infarction or extension of heart muscle disease. In this example, although the muscle remains thickened there is dilatation and poor contraction of the left ventricle.

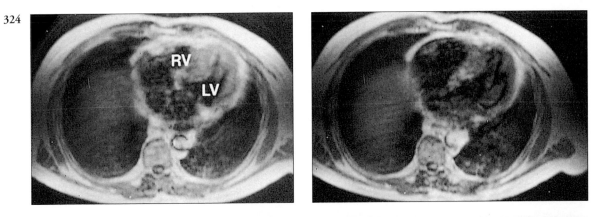

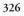

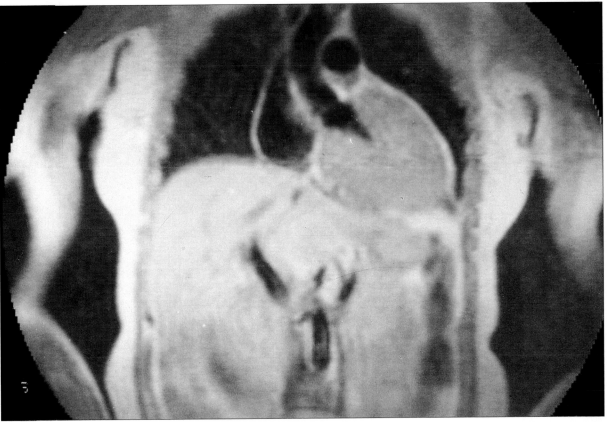

324–326 Magnetic resonance scanning may be useful for defining the extent of left ventricular hypertrophy. A transverse section is shown (systole, **324**; diastole, **325**). There is left ventricular hypertrophy particularly involving the septum and papillary muscles. In a coronal view, severe left ventricular hypertrophy of a concentric nature may also be seen (**326**).

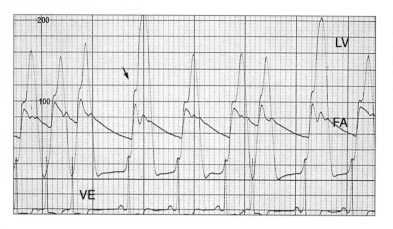

327 Haemodynamic tracing with a resting left ventricular outflow tract gradient with post-extrasystolic potentiation. The ill-sustained pulse in this condition is apparent. Following a ventricular extrasystole (VE) the left ventricular outflow tract gradient increases substantially (arrow).

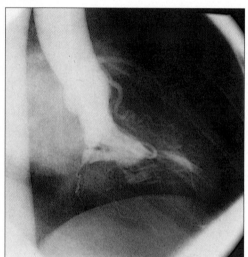

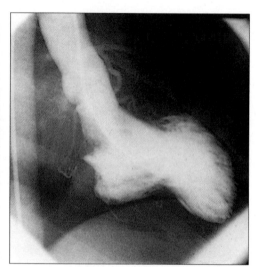

328 & 329 Left ventricular angiogram (systole, **328**; diastole, **329**). There is marked deformation of the left ventricular cavity in this right anterior oblique projection and almost complete mid-cavity elimination and mitral regurgitation into an enlarged atrium.

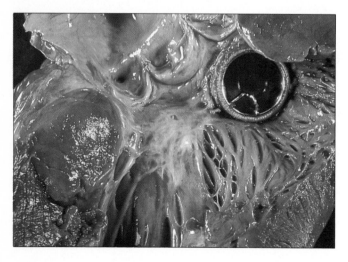

330 Surgery in hypertrophic cardiomyopathy is usually reserved for patients who have a significant resting or provokable left ventricular outflow tract gradient and the symptoms of angina pectoris or heart failure. Mitral regurgitation, if severe, may require a valve replacement. The pathological specimen shows a Björk–Shiley mitral valve replacement in hypertrophic cardiomyopathy. Following myotomy–myectomy, the electrocardiogram often shows a left bundle branch block pattern (**313**). The left ventricle may become dilated and contract less well. Heart failure is not uncommon following a myotomy–myectomy operation.

Restrictive cardiomyopathy

Restrictive cardiomyopathy is characterized by a restriction of diastolic filling due to endocardial and/or a myocardial lesion. Restrictive cardiomyopathies are uncommon in western countries and the most prevalent of these is amyloid infiltration. World-wide, endomyocardial fibrosis with or without eosinophilia is the most common cause of restriction. The restrictive cardiomyopathies demonstrate impaired diastolic function because of abnormal properties of the ventricular walls, which impede ventricular filling. Contractile function is usually unimpaired. The typical presenting features are breathlessness with ankle or abdominal swelling. Cardiac output is normally low and there is a fourth heart sound. The jugular venous pressure is elevated with evidence of restrictive filling of the right ventricle. Investigation in restrictive cardiomyopathy is directed towards establishing its aetiology and determining the presence of intracavity thrombus which may lead to systemic emboli.

Amyloidosis

Amyloidosis may be familial and associated with a polyneuropathy.

Restrictive cardomyopathy
Myocardial
• infiltrative-Amyloid/sarcoid/Gaucher/Hurlers
• storage diseases-Haemochromatosis/Fabry/ glycogen storage
• non-infiltrative-idiopathic/scleroderma
Endomyocardial
• endomyocardial fibrosis
• hypereosinophilic syndrome
• carcinoid

331 Restrictive cardiomyopathy may be classified into causes involving the myocardium with or without the endocardium.

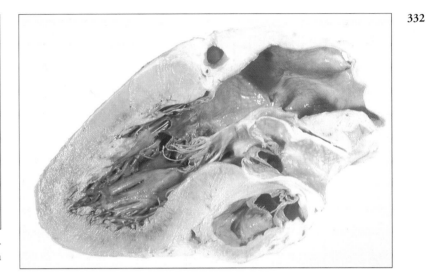

332

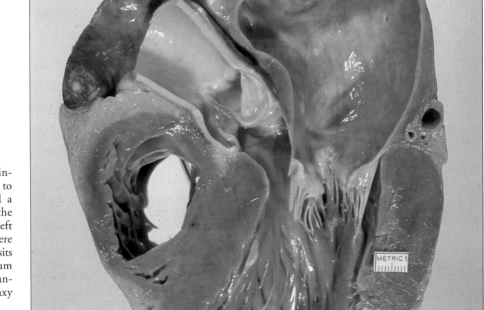

333

332 & 333 Amyloid infiltration of the heart leads to cardiac enlargement and a rubbery consistency of the myocardium (**332**). The left atrium is enlarged and there may be focal amyloid deposits on the mural endocardium which are typically tan-coloured and have a waxy appearance (**333**).

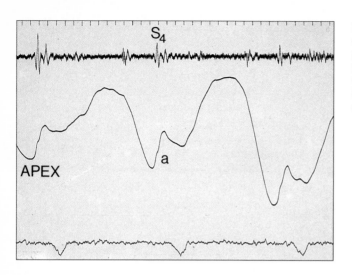

334 The physical signs in amyloid heart disease are dominated by peripheral and abdominal oedema and prominent fourth heart sound (in contrast to constrictive pericarditis). The venous pressure is usually elevated and tends to increase in inspiration (Kussmaul sign). The fourth heart sound may be both heard and felt, as in this example on an indirect apical recording.

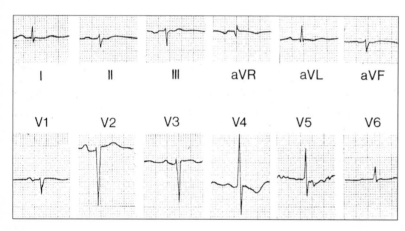

335 The electrocardiogram in amyloid heart disease has a rather characteristic appearance with small QRS voltages often with conduction abnormalities or atrial fibrillation. The low voltages by electrocardiography are in contrast to the echocardiographic appearance of severe left ventricular hypertrophy (see **336 & 337**).

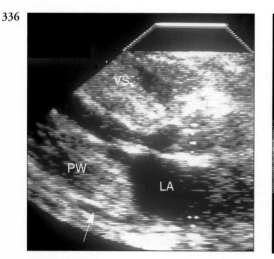
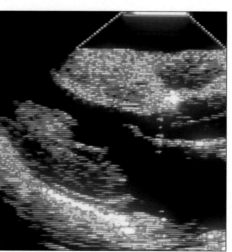

336 & 337 Echocardiogram, parasternal long axis view, in amyloidosis with marked concentric left ventricular hypertrophy and a small posterior pericardial effusion (arrow) (**336**). Colour encoding (**337**) shows that the myocardium reflects echoes with a normal intensity. This is in contrast to most forms of left ventricular hypertrophy where an increased myocardial collagen content leads to an increase in echo amplitude.

338 Magnetic resonance scanning (systole, left; diastole, right) in amyloid heart disease showing thickening of the myocardium with preservation of left ventricular contraction.

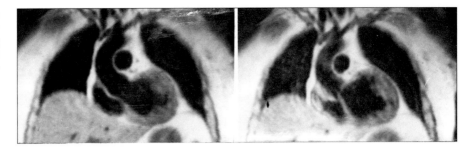

339 Left ventricular pressure trace in amyloid heart disease; there is a raised end-diastolic pressure (LVEDP) with a restricted filling pattern ('dip and plateau').

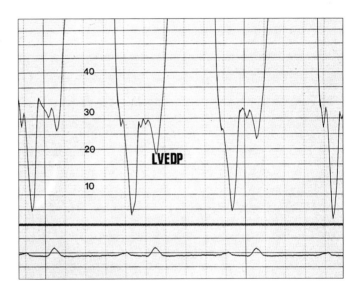

Idiopathic restrictive cardiomyopathy

Idiopathic restrictive cardiomyopathy is an uncommon disorder in the West and often leads to intractable heart failure.

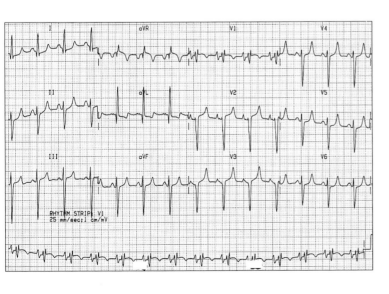

340 The electrocardiogram is non-specific often showing marked atrial enlargement and bundle branch block. In this example, there is a large increase in atrial voltages, left axis deviation and partial right bundle branch block (RSR′ in V1).

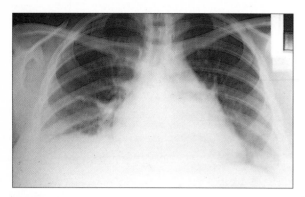

341 Chest radiograph showing mild cardiomegaly and pulmonary venous congestion. There is a linear shadow in the right mid zone with a raised hemi-diaphragm due to a pulmonary embolus.

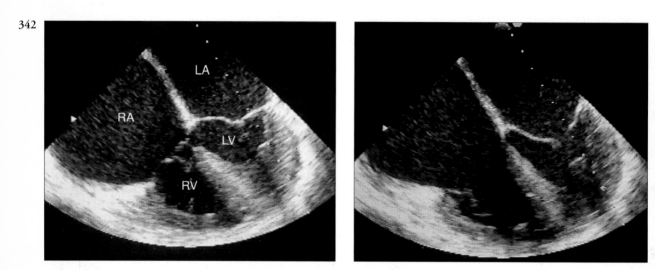

342 & 343 Echocardiogram, transoesophageal long axis, (systole, **342**; diastole, **343**) showing hypertrophied left and right ventricles. Ventricular contraction is unimpaired and there is disproportionate biatrial enlargement due to the abnormal filling properties.

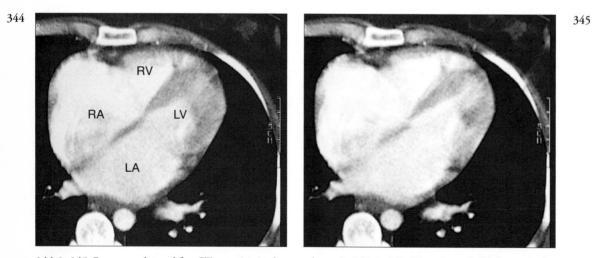

344 & 345 Contrast-enhanced fast CT scanning in the case shown in **342 & 343**. There is marked left ventricular hypertrophy with a small cavity. Biatrial enlargement is seen (systole, **344**; diastole, **345**).

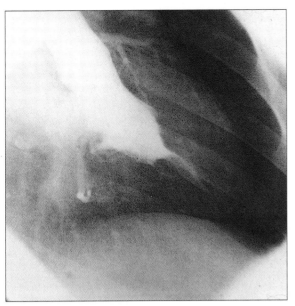 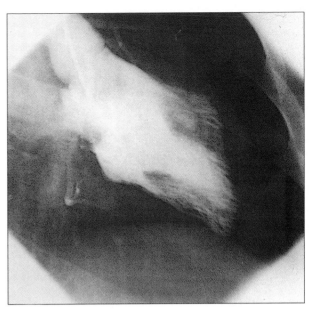

346 & 347 Left ventriculography (systole, **346**; diastole, **347**) in the cases shown in **342–345** showing a hyperdynamic and hypertrophied left ventricle.

Endomyocardial disease

Endomyocardial disease with or without eosinophilia is relatively common in equatorial Africa and is found less commonly in South America, Asia and other non-tropical countries. It is marked by intense endocardial fibrotic thickening of the apex and subvalvular regions of one or both ventricles. It is probable that endomyocardial fibrosis and Löffler endocarditis are different manifestations of the same disease.

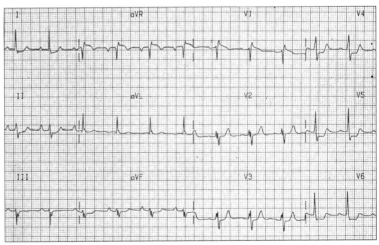

348 The electrocardiogram in eosinophilic heart disease is non-specific. In this example, there is complete right bundle branch block with left axis deviation and widespread ST–T wave changes.

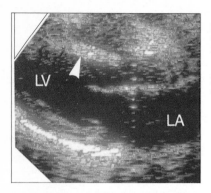

349 Colour encoded echocardiogram, parasternal long axis view, showing bright echoes rising from the myocardium particularly from the ventricular septum (arrow). The bright echoes represent an increase in myocardial collagen and fibrosis (LA left atrium, LV left ventricle).

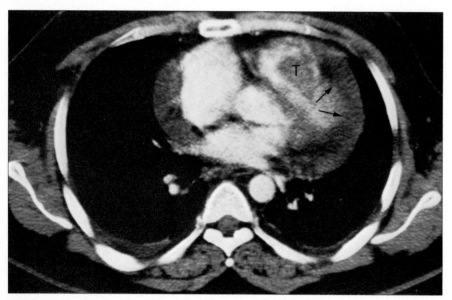

350 Contrast-enhanced computerized tomogram showing intracardiac thrombus (T) in the right ventricle and thickened pericardium (arrows) in endomyocardial disease.

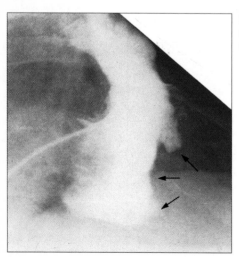

351 Right ventricular angiogram in eosinophilic heart disease showing obliteration of the apex with fibrous tissue (arrows).

Other causes of heart muscle disease

A wide variety of cardiac and systemic diseases may lead to heart failure by the involvement of the myocardium. Most are extremely rare but the following section deals with some of the most frequently encountered conditions.

Sarcoidosis

Sarcoidosis is granulomatous disease of unknown origin with multisystem involvement. While infiltration of the skin, lungs and reticular endothelial system dominates the clinical picture, any tissue can be affected. Cardiac involvement is often not recognized and may occur without other physical findings. Clinical manifestations include left bundle branch or complete heart block, congestive heart failure and ventricular arrhythmias. Most patients develop congestive features but some may present with restrictive signs.

352 The left ventricle and ventricular septum are most commonly affected by sarcoid granulomata (Roberts, 1977).

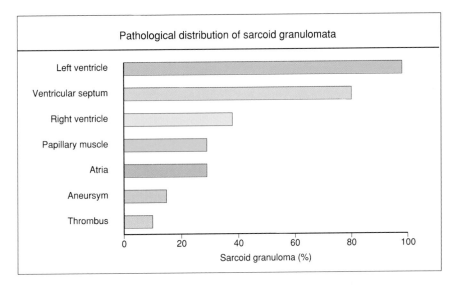

Pathological distribution of sarcoid granulomata

Left ventricle	
Ventricular septum	
Right ventricle	
Papillary muscle	
Atria	
Aneursym	
Thrombus	

Sarcoid granuloma (%)

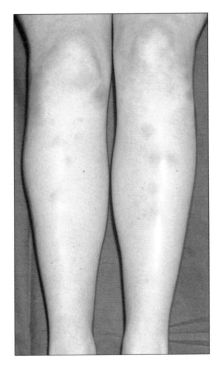

353 Clinical photographs showing erythema nodosum in a patient with sarcoid heart disease and heart failure.

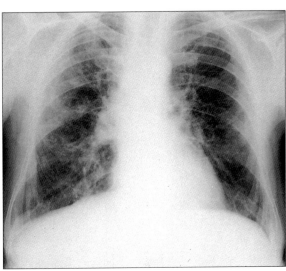

354 Chest radiograph in sarcoidosis. There is fibrosing alveolitis due to sarcoidosis with additional cardiac involvement.

355

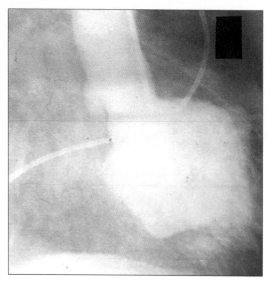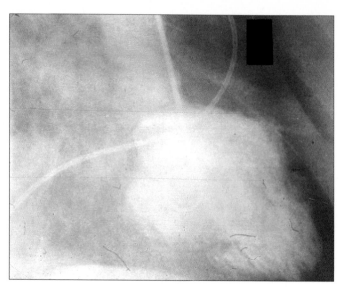

355 & 356 Left ventricular angiogram (systole, **355**; diastole, **356**) showing the characteristic features of cardiac sarcoidosis with basal hypokinesis and preserved apical function.

Neuromuscular diseases

Various neuromuscular diseases may be associated with heart muscle involvement. Heart failure may occur in limb-girdle muscular dystrophy, Friedreich's ataxia, Duchenne's and Becker's muscular dystrophy etc.

357

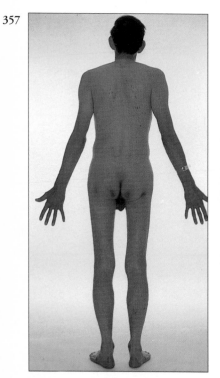

358

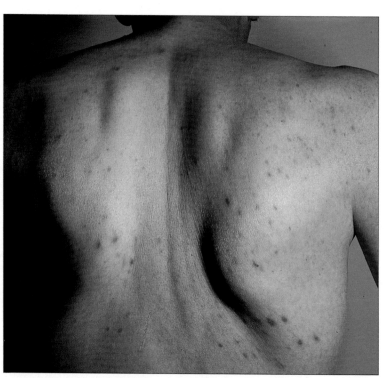

357 & 358 Clinical photographs showing muscle wasting associated with weakness in a patient with skeletal myopathy who had heart muscle disease and failure. In this patient, there was a dilated left ventricle and the ECG showed left bundle branch block.

359 & 360 Becker's, or late onset, and Duchenne's, or early onset muscular dystrophy are frequently associated with cardiac disease (**359**). Shown here is the calf pseudohypertrophy. While the muscular defects are the main limiting factor, death is usually through progressive heart failure. The electrocardiogram in Duchenne's shows a short P–R interval and deep but narrow praecordial Q waves. In this example of Becker's (**360**) there is left ventricular hypertrophy.

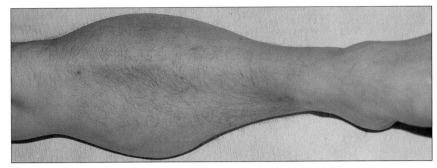

359

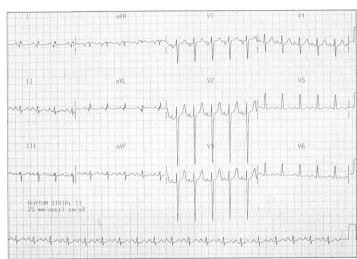

360

361 & 362 Friedreich's ataxia may be associated with heart failure with a hypertrophied or dilated left ventricle. The cardiac involvement is unpredictable and often asymptomatic. There is no relationship between the degree of cardiac and neurological involvement. Clinical photograph of a Friedreich's foot (**361**) showing pes cavus (clawing of the toes is not seen). Kyphoscoliosis commonly accompanies ataxia and muscle weakness. The echocardiogram (**362**), parasternal long axis view, (systole, left; diastole, right) shows septal hypertrophy and ventricular dilatation. The appearances of hypertrophic cardiomyopathy may be observed.

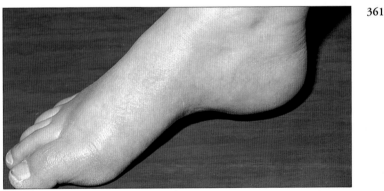

361

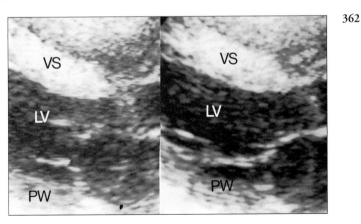

362

363 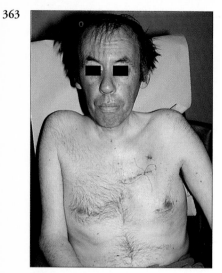 364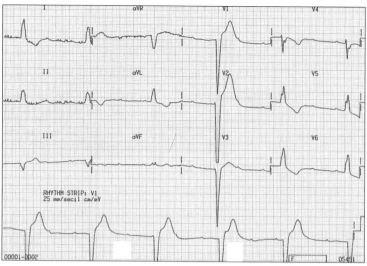

363 & 364 Dystrophia myotonica is a rare autosomal dominant disease most commonly associated with weakness and atrophy of neck muscles. Myotonia is associated with other system features including cataracts, baldness and testicular atrophy. Patients may develop heart failure and conduction system disease. In this case, the typical facies are seen in a patient with heart failure who had recently undergone a pacemaker implantation. The ECG showed complete heart block (**364**).

365   366   367

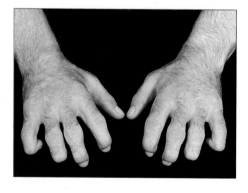

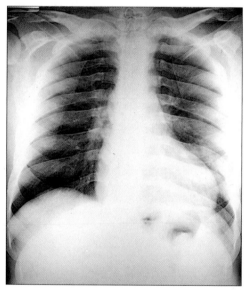

365–367 There are a large number of inborn errors of metabolism that have a direct or secondary effect on the heart. They are all very rare and few lead to heart failure; mucopolysaccharidosis, Fabry's disease, haemochromatosis and the glycogen storage disorders are the most common of these. Short stature, coarse features, corneal clouding, skeletal deformity and mental retardation are common, as seen here in a case of Hurler's syndrome (**365 & 366**). There is mild cardiomegaly and the ribs are broad and spatulate (**367**). Valve disease and pseudohypertrophy of the myocardium are frequently seen and may lead to heart failure.

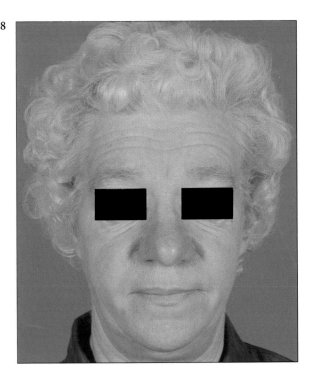

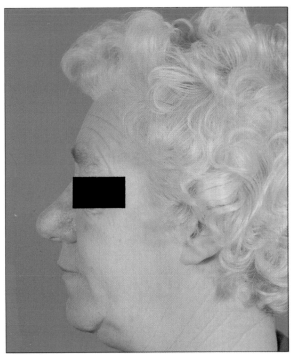

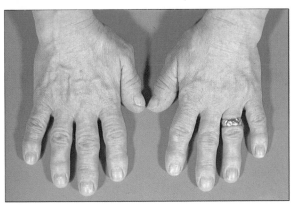

368–371 Endocrine disorders may affect the myocardium and lead to heart failure. The most common of these are acromegaly and phaeochromocytoma but hyperthyroidism and Cushing's syndrome may occasionally lead to heart failure. Heart failure develops in acromegaly due to hypertension, diabetes, coronary disease and possibly a specific myocardial disease. The facial appearances are typical with a prominent mandible and overgrowth of the frontal ridges (**368 & 369**). The hands may become broad and spade-like (**370**). Enlargement of the pituitary gland (arrow) is best seen by contrast-enhanced CT scanning (**371**). The cardiac features are non-specific with a dilated and poorly-contracting hypertrophied left ventricle.

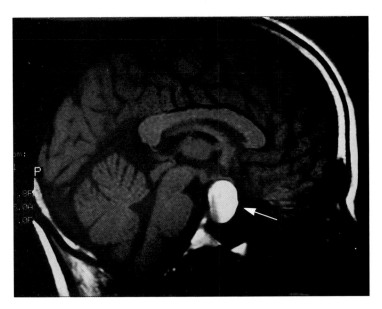

372

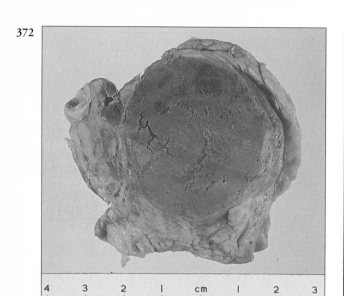

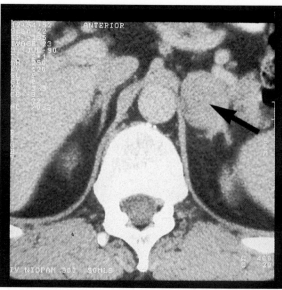

374

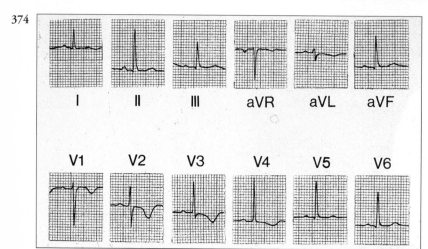

372–374 Phaeochromocytoma may present with a constellation of signs and symptoms, paroxysmal hypertension being the most common. Heart failure may ensue due to hypertension (often malignant grade) or a catecholamine induced cardiomyopathy. Gross pathology of a formalin-fixed adrenal phaeochromocytoma (**372**). The site of the tumour is best demonstrated by CT scanning (arrow, **373**). The ECG may show left ventricular hypertrophy or deep symmetrical T wave inversion due to catecholamine cardiomyopathy (**374**).

5. HYPERTENSION

Hypertension is an important cause of heart failure, particularly in association with coronary heart disease. While the Framingham study showed that hypertension was statistically very important in the aetiology of heart failure, with the widespread treatment of elevated blood pressure in the last few decades it has become less common.

Hypertensive heart failure usually presents with dilated and hypertrophied left ventricle but occasionally the heart size may be normal and there is severe concentric hypertrophy. In the latter circumstances, the mechanism of heart failure is similar to that seen in hypertrophic cardiomyopathy with impaired diastolic function. Most cases of hypertension causing heart failure are of unknown aetiology but any secondary cause of hypertension may be responsible.

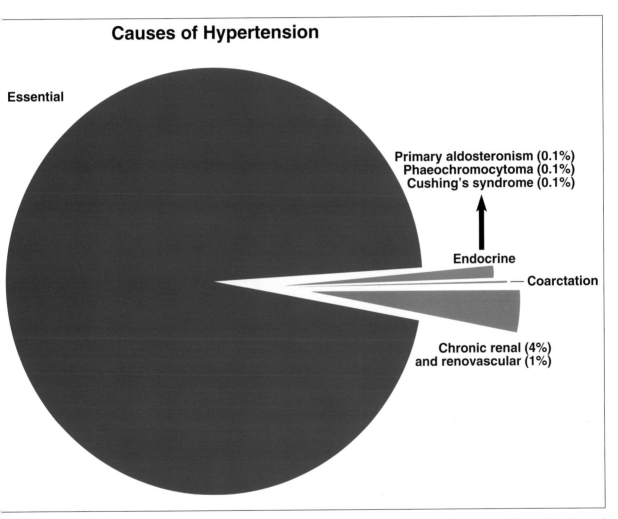

375 The vast majority of cases of hypertension are of essential or idiopathic origin. Coarctation of the aorta, endocrine disorders and renal disease account for approximately 5 per cent of causes.

376

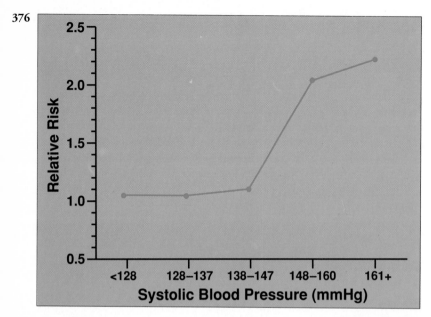

377

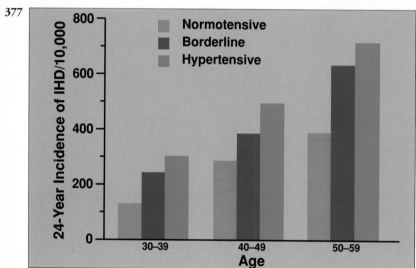

376–378 Hypertension may lead to the development of heart failure by accelerated coronary artery disease or pressure overload alone. The relative risk of developing coronary artery disease increases rapidly in patients with blood pressure exceeding 138–147 mmHg (**376**), and this applies in all age groups (**377**). The effect of hypertension on the development of coronary disease is additive with other risk factors (**378**). Patients with established and even borderline hypertension are at increased risk of developing heart failure (**379**).

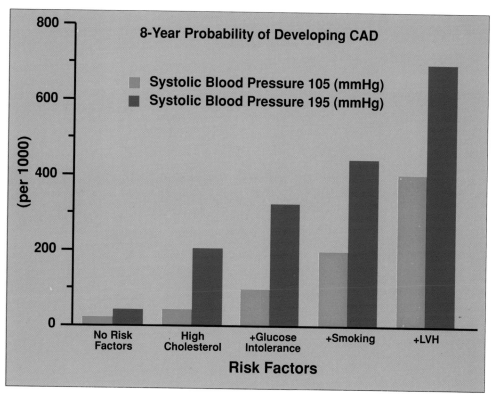

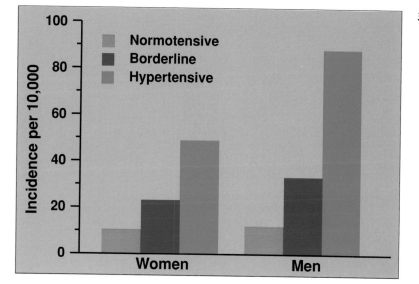

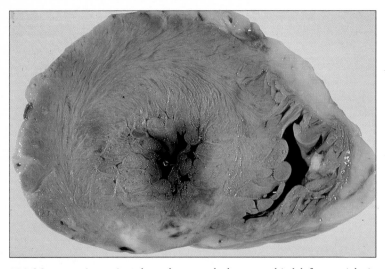

380 Macroscopic section through a grossly hypertrophied left ventricle in hypertensive heart failure.

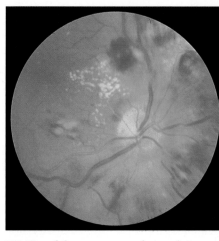

381 Heart failure occurs more frequently in sever hypertension particularly in the malignant o accelerated phase. Retinal fundus showing extensive areas of haemorrhage and exudate papilloedema may be noted with raised opti fundus, haemorrhages and exudates.

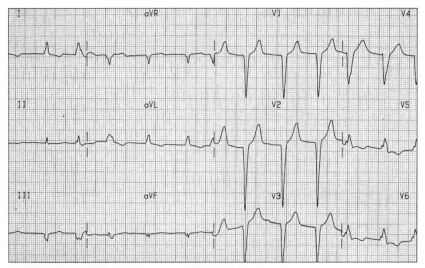

382 The electrocardiogram in hyper tensive heart disease may show lef ventricular hypertrophy with a strain pattern or, alternatively, left bundl branch block as in this example. Th development of atrial fibrillation, as seer here, is a common sequela and may lea to heart failure.

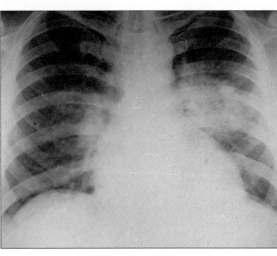

383 The chest radiograph in hypertensive heart disease may show normally sized heart, as in this case, or cardiomegaly. There is sever pulmonary oedema.

384 Echocardiogram (parasternal short axis view, left; long axis view, right) in a patient with hypertensive heart failure with a hypertrophied left ventricle (LV) and posterior pericardial effusion (PE); (LA left atrium; RV right ventricle).

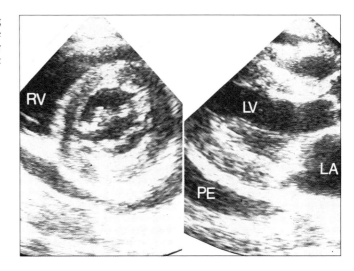

385 & 386 Magnetic resonance images, transverse section, (systole, **385**; diastole, **386**) in a patient with severe concentric ventricular hypertrophy due to hypertension.

385

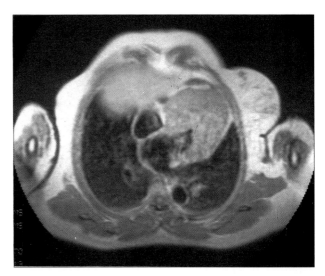

386

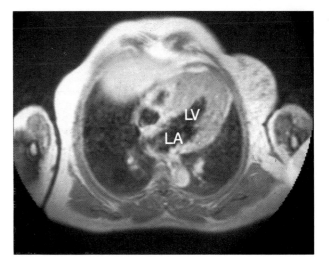

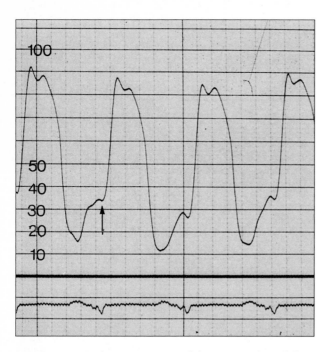

387 Pressure recording in a patient with hypertensive heart failure. The left ventricular end-diastolic pressure (arrow) is markedly elevated at 35 mmHg. With the onset of heart failure, the systolic arterial pressure may fall towards the normal range.

6. PERICARDIAL DISEASE

Constriction

Acute pericarditis is characterized by chest pain, a pericardial friction rub and electrocardiographic abnormalities. Pericarditis may be clinically unapparent and only very rarely does the acute syndrome lead to heart failure; however, breathlessness is quite a common presenting feature. Constrictive pericarditis was first described in 1842 and may present when a fibrotic, thickened and adherent pericardium restricts diastolic filling. In an initial episode of acute pericarditis, there may be fibrin deposits and a pericardial effusion. Then comes a subacute stage of organization and re-absorption of the effusion. In the chronic stage, there will be fibrous thickening of the pericardium with loss of pericardial space. The rate of progression from the acute to chronic stage is very variable and depends upon the underlying disease aetiology. In the past, tuberculosis was the leading cause of pericarditis, and is still found in the developing countries. Constriction may follow many years after irradiation, especially for breast cancer or Hodgkin's disease.

Causes of pericarditis
Idiopathic
Connective tissue disease SLE/RF/RA/Takayasu's/PAN/Wegeners
Uraemia and haemodialysis
Acute bacterial
Trauma
Tuberculosis
Fungal infections
Radiation
Drugs Hydrallazine/procainamide/penicillin, etc.
Aortic dissection
Chylopericardium
Viral disease
Dressler's and post MI syndomes
Sarcoidosis/amyloid/pancreatitis/EMF/myoedema

388 Acute pericarditis may be idiopathic or due to bacterial infection, myocardial infarction, trauma and many other causes.

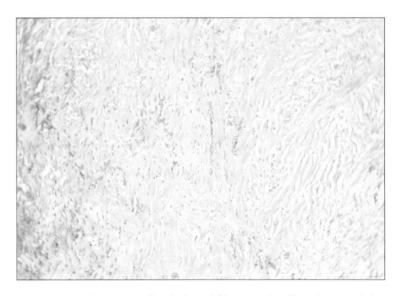

389 Microscopic section of a thickened fibrous pericardium in constrictive pericarditis.

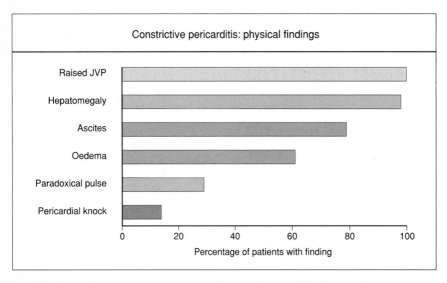

Constrictive pericarditis: physical findings

390 The physical signs in constrictive pericarditis are dominated by the raised venous pressure and hepatomegaly, ascites and peripheral oedema. Pulsus paradoxus and a pericardial knock, although pathognomonic, are less commonly seen (Fowler *et al.*,1985).

391

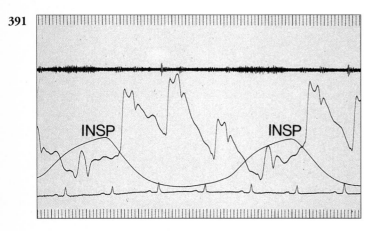

392

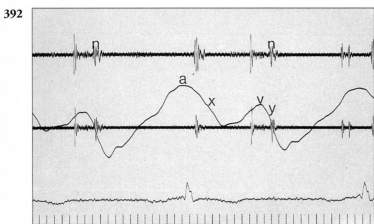

391 & 392 Pulsus paradoxus, which is not paradoxical but is an increase in the normal physiological response to respiration, is shown by a marked fall in the pulse volume and duration during inspiration here shown on an indirect pulse recording (**391**). Constrictive pericarditis restricts right ventricular filling causing a rapid Y descent in the venous pressure which will be coincidental with the pericardial knock (n) (**392**).

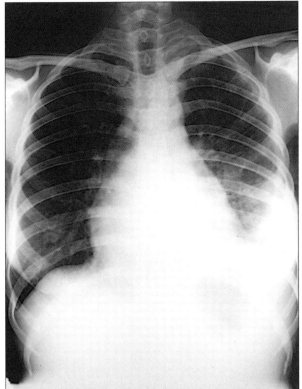

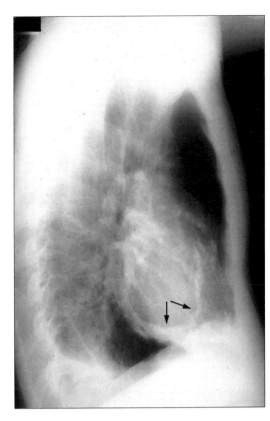

393 & 394 The chest radiograph in acute tuberculous pericarditis in this example shows cardiomegaly due to a pericardial effusion and a left pleural effusion(**393**). In chronic constriction, the pericardium is often calcified; here shown on a lateral radiograph (arrows) (**394**).

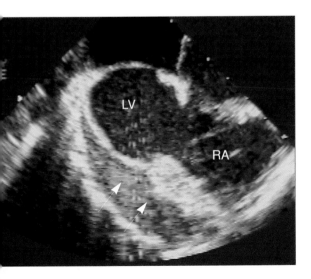

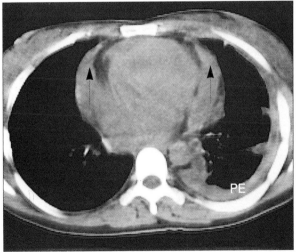

395 The pericardium, even when markedly thickened, may be difficult to image by transthoracic echocardiography. Transoesophageal echocardiography may allow an anatomical diagnosis to be made. In this case of tuberculosis the pericardium is very thick, overlying the right atrioventricular groove (arrows). (Same case as is shown in **393**).

396 CT scanning will define thickened pericardium (arrows) in this example of tuberculosis with a left pleural effusion (PE), the same case as is shown in **393** and **395**.

397

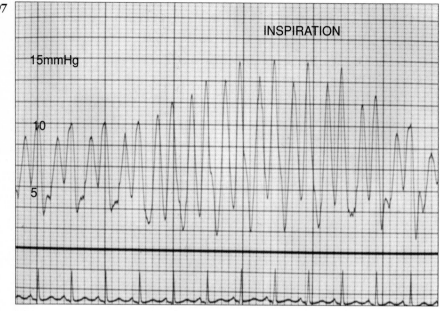

398

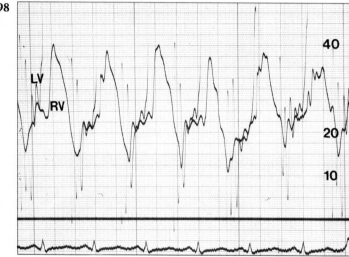

397 & 398 There is a marked increase in right atri[al] pressure on inspiration (this is equivalent to the Kussma[ul] sign). Simultaneous right ventricular and left ventricul[ar] pressure with equalization of both end-diastolic pressur[es] and also a 'dip and plateau' in the pressure wave for[m] (**398**).

Cardiac tamponade

Intrapericardial pressure is normally close to intrapleural pressure and lower than right and left ventricular diastolic pressures. Increase in the intrapericardial pressure, secondary to fluid accumulation, leads to cardiac tamponade, characterized by elevation of intracardiac pressures, pro[g]ressive limitation of diastolic filling and reduction in strok[e] volume. Cardiac tamponade may occur from any cause [of] pericarditis and may occur in acute or chronic forms.

Causes of cardiac tamponade

Malignant

Idiopathic

Trauma
Dresslers

Uraemic

SLE
Myxoedema

Aneurysm

Anticoag (MI/DCM)

Radiation

Bacterial

Iatrogenic

399 The aetiology of cardiac tamponade may be idiopathic or from malignant disease and a large number of other causes.

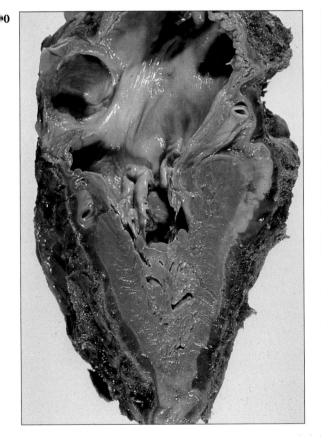

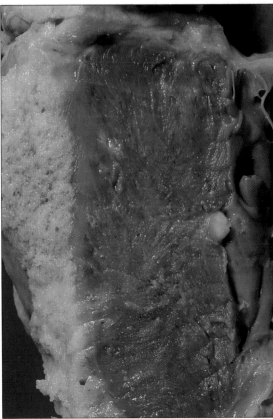

400 & 401 Pathological specimens demonstrating pericardial disease. In a patient with sepsis and liver failure, the heart is surrounded by adherent fibrin and is stained diffusely green from bilirubin (**400**). Macroscopic view of the left ventricular wall in a patient with fungal septicaemia; there is a thick white fibrin exudate of pericarditis (**401**).

402

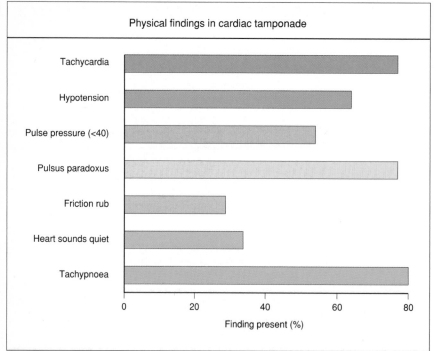

Physical findings in cardiac tamponade

Finding present (%)

- Tachycardia
- Hypotension
- Pulse pressure (<40)
- Pulsus paradoxus
- Friction rub
- Heart sounds quiet
- Tachypnoea

403

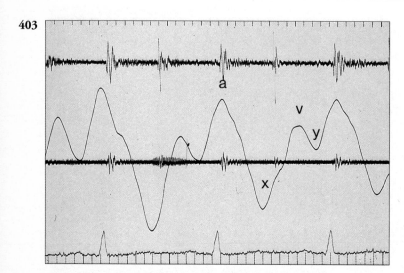

402 & 403 The physical signs in tamponade are dominated by tachycardia, low blood pressure and pulsus paradoxus (**402**, Fowler *et al.*, 1984). Cardiac tamponade may be differentiated from constrictive pericarditis, as a rapid x descent is dominant in the venous pressure (here shown on an indirect recording(**403**).

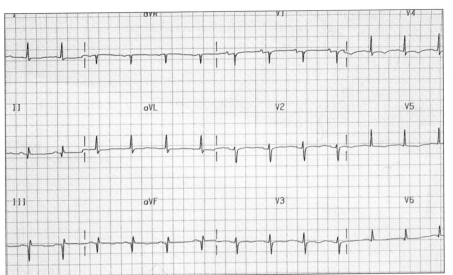

404

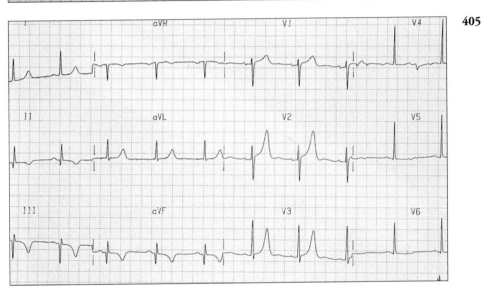

405

404 & 405 The electrocardiogram in tamponade often has small QRS voltages (**404**). Following aspiration of the pericardial effusion and relief of tamponade, QRS voltages return to normal (**405**).

406

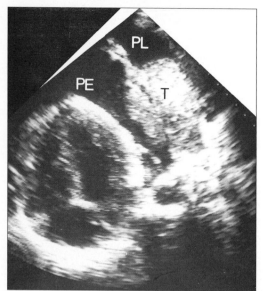

407

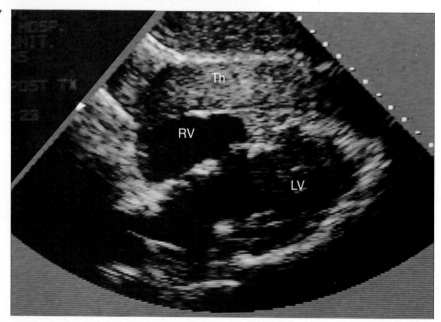

406 & 407 Echocardiography may demonstrate the cause of cardiac tamponade. A pleural effusion (PL) and pericardial effusion (PE) due to a pericardial tumour may lead to tamponade. The tumour (T) can be seen attached to the pericardium (**406**). Cardiac tamponade may occur post cardiac surgery with blood and thrombus accumulation in the pericardial space. A subcostal view showing anterior thrombus (Th) (**407**).

7. INFECTION AND HEART FAILURE

Infective endocarditis

All forms of infection may precipitate heart failure in a patient with impaired cardiac function or valve disease. However, infective endocarditis may rapidly destroy cardiac valves and lead to acute and chronic heart failure. Severe regurgitation may occur even when, initially, only mild valvar abnormalities are present. Rarely, vegetations may produce stenosis. The diagnosis of infective endocarditis must also be considered in any patient who presents with non-specific symptoms of pyrexia and who has underlying valve lesions. With the development of severe regurgitation, heart failure may develop rapidly. The nature of infective endocarditis has changed over the past few decades with the decline in the incidence of rheumatic heart disease and an increase in the abuse of parenteral drugs and the involvement of prosthetic heart valves. Most patients have some underlying heart disease and, at present, mitral valve prolapse is numerically the most common.

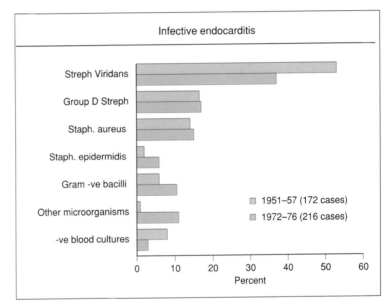

408 In the past few decades, *Streptococcus viridans* sp. has become a less common cause of endocarditis but still remains the most frequent organism isolated (Wilson *et al.*, 1977).

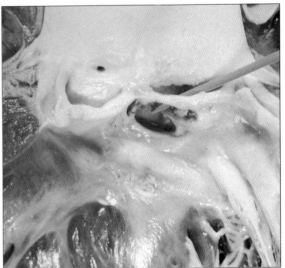

409 Destruction of a cusp, in this case a bicuspid aortic valve, will lead to acute valvar regurgitation and heart failure.

410

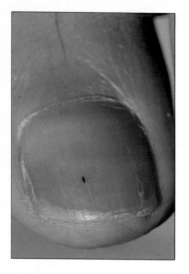

411

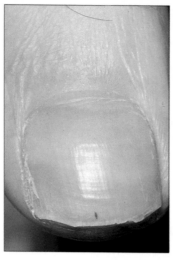

412

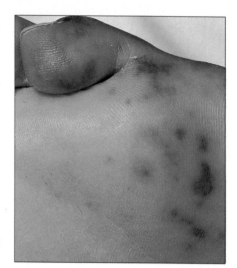

413

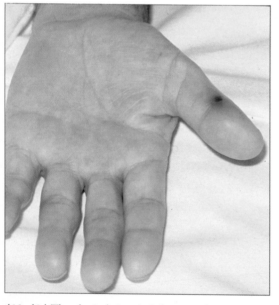

414

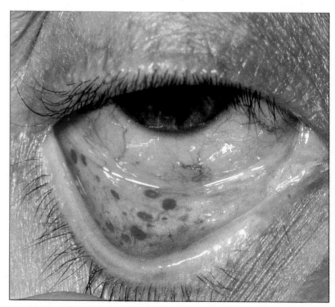

410–414 The physical signs in infective endocarditis include splinter haemorrhages (shown early in **410**, and growing out in **411**), dermal infarcts which may occur from septic emboli (**412**), Osler's nodes (**413**) and subconjunctival haemorrhage (**414**).

415

415–421 Echocardiography may determine the presence of a valvar vegetation which will be present in the majority of cases with infective endocarditis. A mobile vegetation is seen (arrow) (415) attached to the anterior leaflet of the mitral valve. During the cardiac cycle, the vegetation prolapses into the left ventricular outflow tract. The vegetation may form on ruptured mitral valve chordae and prolapse backwards in to the left atrium (arrow) (416–418). Transoesophageal echocardiography considerably increases the sensitivity of the diagnosis of vegetations, which may have important clinical implications. A small vegetation on the aortic valve not seen by transthoracic imaging is shown, attached to the ventricular aspect of the valve (arrow) associated with severe regurgitation as a turbulent jet, by colour flow Doppler (∗) (419–421).

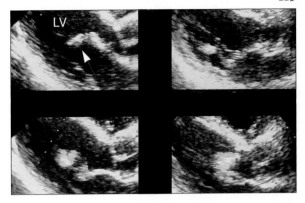

416   **417**   **418**

419   **420**   **421**

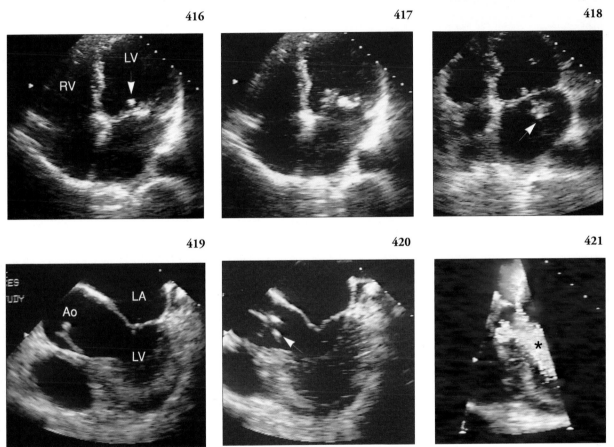

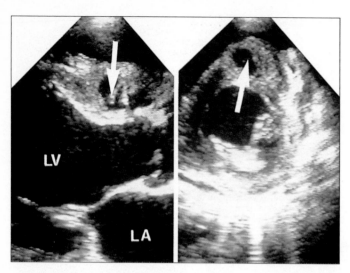

422 The development of an aortic root abscess is a potentially lethal complication of endocarditis and may lead to widespread destruction of the valves and conducting system. A septal abscess arising from aortic infection extends downwards into the septum (**422**). Shown in the aortic root (arrow) in the parasternal long axis view (left) and extending downwards in the left ventricle on a short axis view (arrow, right).

423

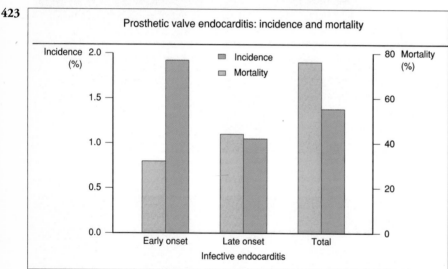

423 & 424 Infection of prosthetic heart valves accounts for 5–15 per cent of all cases. The risk of endocarditis peaks in the weeks after surgery and thereafter remains stable at a much lower risk rate. Both early and late endocarditis carry a very poor prognosis (**423**, Wilson *et al.*, 1982). The organisms involved differ in the early and late forms but most confer a high mortality (**424**, Wilson *et al.*, 1977).

424

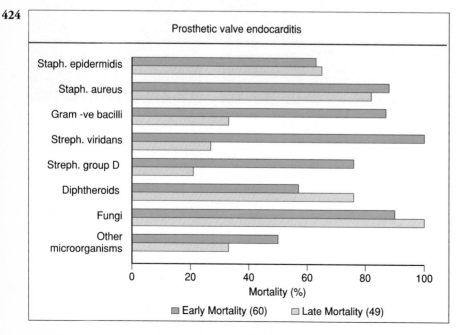

425

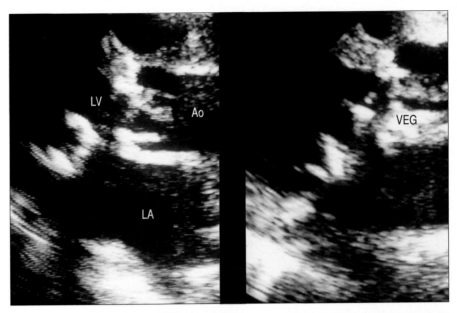

426

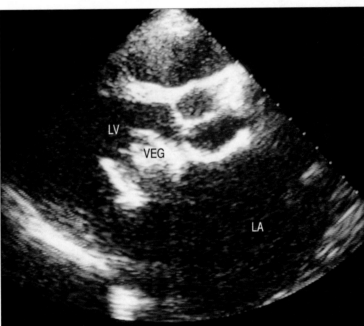

425 & 426 Echocardiography may be able to detect the presence of valvar infection by the presence of vegetations. Here (**425**) the vegetation involves the aortic xenograft and extends up the ascending aorta. Echocardiography may also reveal destruction of a mitral xenograph (leading to severe regurgitation), disruption of the sewing ring and valvar obstruction (**426**).

8. CARDIAC TUMOURS

Cardiac tumours, particularly myxomata, can produce a broad spectrum of cardiac and non-cardiac findings including fever, cachexia and malaise as well as systemic and pulmonary emboli. Left atrial tumours are usually pedunculated and mobile and prolapse into the mitral orifice resulting in obstruction to atrioventricular blood flow as well as mitral regurgitation. The resultant signs and symptoms often mimic mitral valve disease with orthopnoea, paroxysmal nocturnal dyspnoea, pulmonary oedema, cough, chest pains and fatigue. There may well be systemic features and the symptoms may be related to the patient's body position. Tumours may present with disturbances of conduction or cardiac rhythm, particularly if they involve the atrioventricular node. Right atrial tumours are much less common and may present with right heart failure. Primary tumours of the heart are rare and the diagnosis is best made by echocardiography or magnetic resonance scanning.

427 The incidence of cardiac tumours: more than a third of the total are myomata; most other tumours of the heart are of connective tissue origin (myxomata) and benign (Urba, 1986).

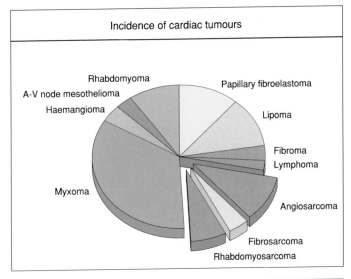

428 The frequency distribution of atrial and ventricular myxomata. Most frequently these arise in the left atrium and much less commonly in the right atrium and the ventricles (Goldman *et al.*, 1986).

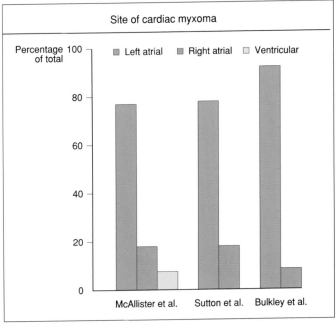

429

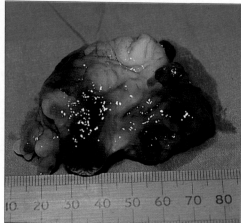

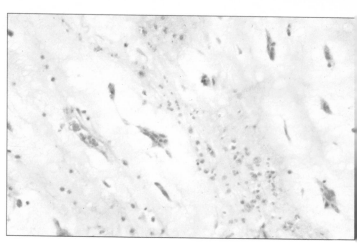

429 & 430 The pathological features of myxomata are variable. The tumour is heterogeneous with islands of mucoid material and haemorrhage. Such tumours obstruct the mitral valve and may lead to heart failure; a surgically resected left atrial myxoma is shown (**429**). On microscopy, a myxoma shows a weakly eosinophilic and basophilic matrix (**430**).

431

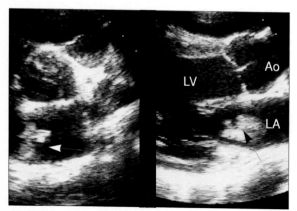

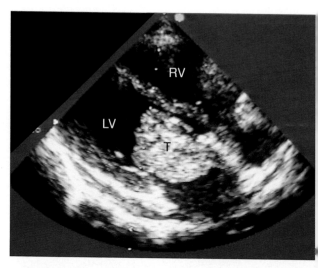

431 & 432 Echocardiograms in left atrial myxomata. In a parasternal long axis view (**431**) a small tumour is seen in the left atrium; it is seen attached to the intra-atrial septum (left, **431**). A large heterogeneous mass in the left atrium may obstruct the mitral orifice and lead to heart failure (**432**). The tumour (T) is attached by a pedicle to the interatrial septum in the region of the foramen ovale.

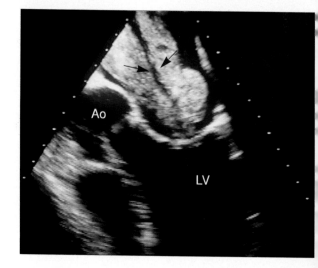

432b Transoesophageal echocardiography will more precisely define the anatomy of an atrial myxoma and site of attachment. A cleft left atrial myxoma is seen filling the atrial cavity (arrow).

9. CONGENITAL HEART DISEASE

During the last few decades many patients have reached adult life with cardiac malformations which are uncorrected or only partially surgically corrected. Most forms of congenital heart disease do not lead to heart failure except by the development of pulmonary hypertension or by deterioration in cardiac function. The presence of a large left-to-right shunt (as in an atrial and ventricular septal defect) may also lead to heart failure. By inducing pressure overload, congenital valve disease (see **180**) and coarctation of the aorta may also lead to heart failure.

Atrial septal defect

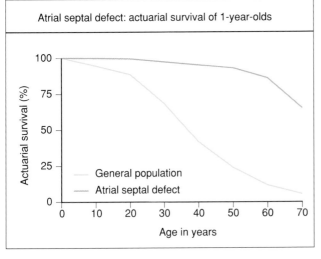

433 The actuarial survival for atrial septal defects and the general population is shown. Until early middle age, there is little impairment in prognosis. Mortality then remains considerably elevated throughout the following decades. (Campbell *et al.*, 1970).

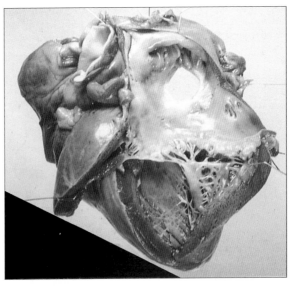

434 Secundum atrial septal defect view from the right side. There is dilatation of the right ventricle and atrium.

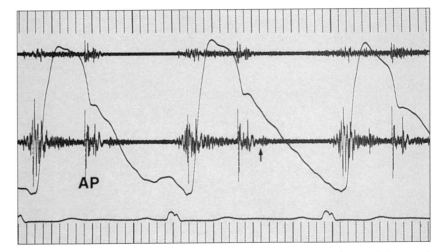

435 The physical signs in atrial septal defect are dominated by fixed splitting of the second heart sound, shown here by phonocardiography. In large defects, there may be a tricuspid flow murmur and a right ventricular third heart sound (arrow) as well as an ejection systolic murmur.

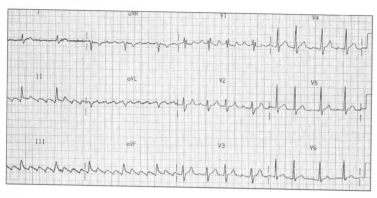

436 Electrocardiogram in secundum atrial septal defect showing atrial flutter and right bundle branch block. The axis is towards the right, in contrast to primum defects where it is towards the left. The development of atrial fibrillation and flutter in atrial septal defect often causes haemodynamic deterioration.

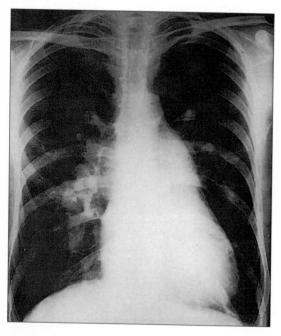

437 The chest radiograph in atrial septal defect with heart failure showing cardiomegaly, dilatation of the pulmonary arteries and pulmonary plethora.

438

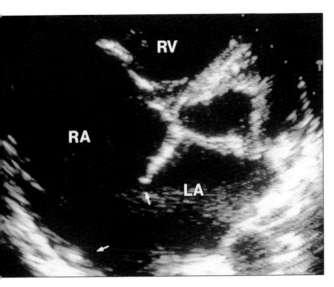

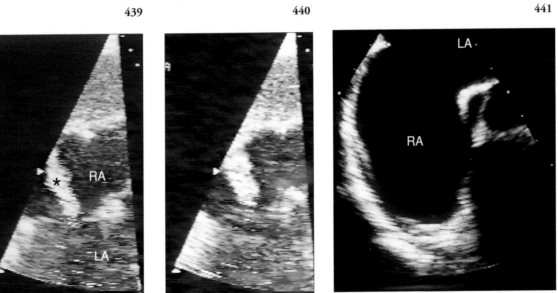

438–441 Echocardiography is the method of choice for diagnosing the presence and haemodynamic significance of atrial septal defects. The atrial septum is deficient in the secundum portion (arrows) and there is dilatation of the right atrium representing a significant left-to-right shunt (**438**). A primum atrial septal defect will be seen higher in the septum. Colour flow Doppler demonstrates a narrow (**439**) and then widening (**440**) turbulent jet of blood flow (∗) crossing the atrial septum from the left to right atrium in this subcostal view. This technique will demonstrate small defects and patency of the foramen ovale. Trans-oesophageal echocardiography may be useful for studying the anatomy of the interatrial septum; in this example, the septum is deficient with considerable right atrial enlargement (**441**).

439   **440**   **441**

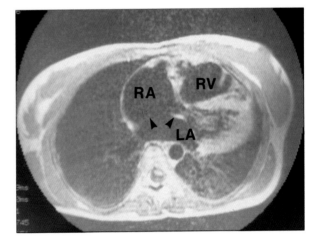

442 Magnetic resonance scanning in a secundum atrial septal defect with enlargement of the right atrium and ventricle.

Ventricular septal defect

Small ventricular septal defects are usually asymptomatic. However, pulmonary hypertension and impaired ventricular function in large defects may result in right heart failure.

443

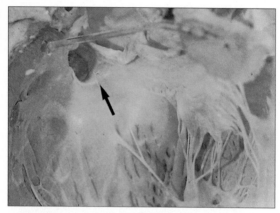

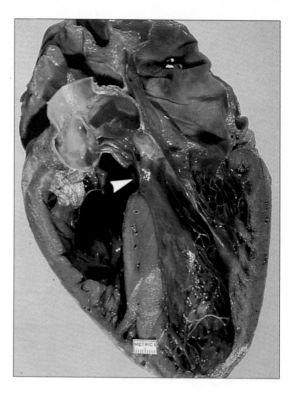

443 & 444 A subaortic ventricular septal defect (arrow) is shown in the opened left ventricle (**443**). This defect is relatively small, unlike that seen in **444**, which is a large defect with dilated left and right ventricles and pulmonary hypertension.

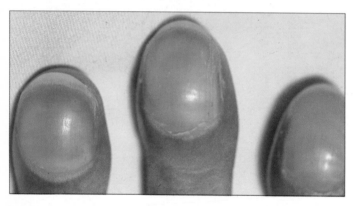

445 In a pulmonary hypertensive patient with ventricular septal defect cyanosis may be seen around th lips and there may be clubbing of the fingers and toe Severe clubbing leads to a drumstick type appearance the fingers.

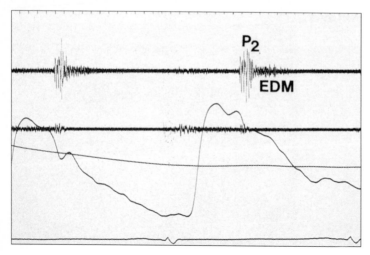

446 The physical findings in pulmonary hypertensiv ventricular septal defect are dominated by a lou pulmonary closure sound, right ventricular cardia impulse and the stigmata of right heart failure. Th murmur may remain evident with a loud secon sound; however, when there is equalization of th right and left ventricular pressures, the murmur abolished, pulmonary closure is loud (P_2) and ther will be an early diastolic murmur of secondar pulmonary regurgitation.

447 The electrocardiogram in a ventricular septal defect with pulmonary hypertension shows gross right ventricular hypertrophy right axis deviation and very tall r waves with deep s waves in v5–6).

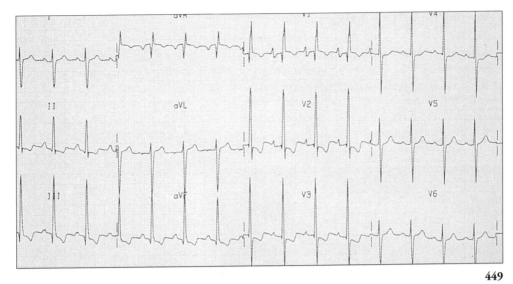

449

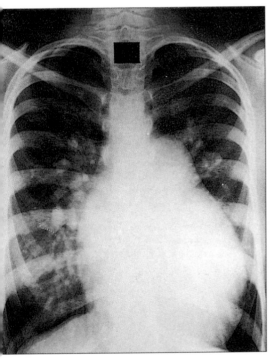

448 Chest radiograph of a small ventricular defect will be normal, but large pulmonary hypertensive ventricular septal defects lead to cardiomegaly, prominence of the pulmonary artery and pulmonary plethora.

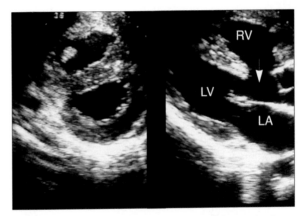

450

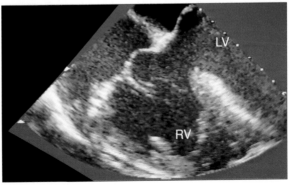

449 & 450 The echocardiogram may delineate the site and size of the septal defect. A parasternal long axis view (right) and short axis view (left) of a large subaortic ventricular septal defect (arrow); the right ventricle is enlarged and hypertrophied (**449**). Colour flow Doppler imaging will localize the site of a ventricular septal defect. This is particularly important in small defects which are difficult to image. Transoesophageal echocardiography may yield information on the nature of the ventricular septal defect; in this case it is the ventricular component of an atrioventricular septal defect (**450**).

Coarctation of the aorta

Coarctation of the aorta is a congenital narrowing of the upper portion of the ascending aorta at the site of the arterial duct. It is slightly more common in males than females, and accounts for up to 5 per cent of congenital heart lesions. Presentation may be a neonatal life with heart failure, but the condition may also be diagnosed in adults who are completely asymptomatic. The physical signs in th adult are hypertension in the upper body and weak, delayed lower limb pulses; collateral murmurs may be present ove the back. Patients may present in adult life with hyper tension, cardiac failure, endocarditis, aortic rupture an intracranial lesions.

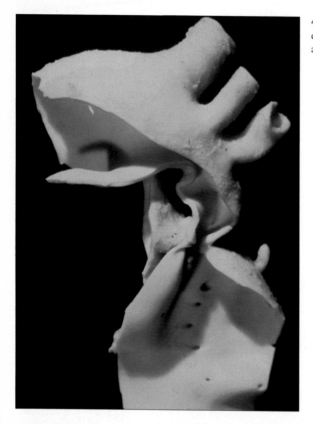

451 Pathological specimen showing an aortic coarctation. There is discrete shelf-like narrowing of the aorta below the left subclavia artery.

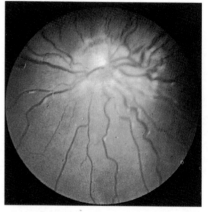

452 Retinal photograph showing tortuous vessels which reflect both the hypertension and also the tortuosity that occurs in upper limb vessels.

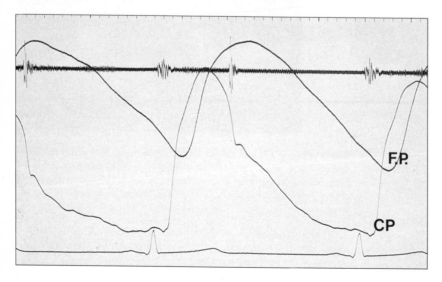

453 Examination of the pulses i coarctation (here shown as indirec recordings) reveals that the femora pulse is both delayed and weak whe compared to the carotid pulse.

454 & 455 The electrocardiogram may be normal or show the voltage criteria for left ventricular hypertrophy (**454**). Five years later, this patient presented with heart failure; the trace now shows an increased QRS voltage, lateral ST segment depression and T wave inversion (**455**).

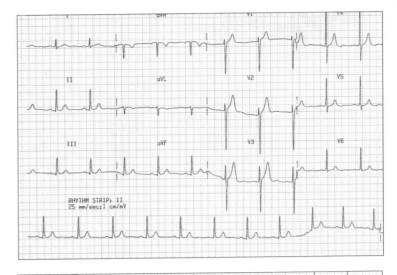

454

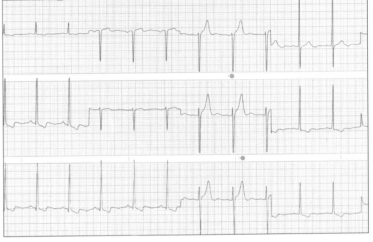

455

456 & 457 A chest radiography classically shows rib notching (arrow); the heart size may be normal (**456**) or may be enlarged (**457**). Pulmonary oedema occurs as a late phenomenon as a consequence of hypertension and associated aortic valve disease.

456

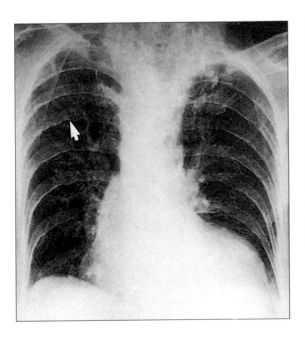

457

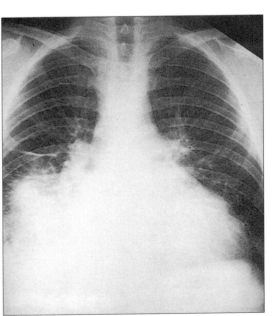

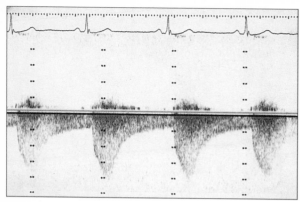

458 Continuous Doppler wave recording from the suprasternal notch showing a peak velocity in systole of almost 4 m/s across the aortic coarctation. This equates to a gradient of approximately 60 mmHg. Throughout diastole, there remains a gradient across this area representing continuous flow.

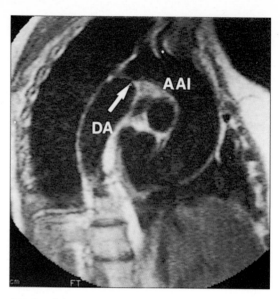

459 In adults, it is usually not possible to demonstrate coarctation by echocardiography. However, magnetic resonance imaging, here showing transverse sections, will demonstrate the site of the obstruction (arrow). The ascending aorta (AAI) is dilated, the descending aorta (DA) is of normal size.

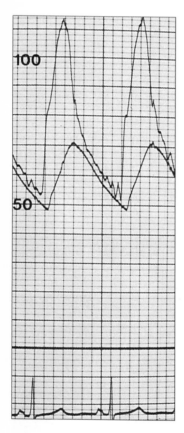

460 Aortic and femoral artery pressure demonstrating the gradient across the coarctation.

10. PULMONARY HYPERTENSION

Pulmonary hypertension of any cause may eventually lead to the development of right heart failure and is associated with a poor prognosis. The normal mean pulmonary artery pressure is 6–10 mmHg and hypertension is diagnosed when the pressure reaches 20 mmHg. Heart failure develops due to impairment of ventricular contraction and tricuspid regurgitation. Primary pulmonary hypertension is the commonest cause of heart failure but chronic lung disease, chronically raised left atrial pressure (as in mitral valve disease), Eisenmenger's syndrome, collagen vascular disease and hypoventilation may also be responsible.

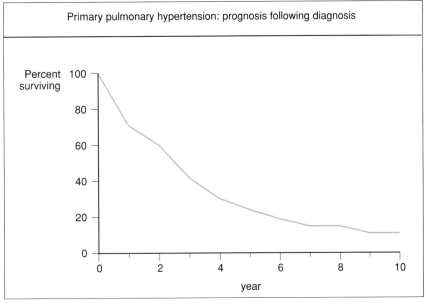

461 The prognosis following the diagnosis of primary pulmonary hypertension is very poor with less than 25 per cent of patients surviving five years (Fuster *et al*).

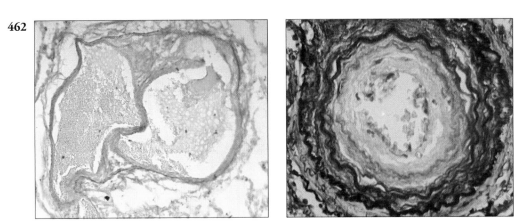

462 & 463 Microscopic section of the lung in thromboembolic disease causing pulmonary hypertension with grade IV arteriolar dilatation (**462**). Histology of the pulmonary artery shows splitting of the internal elastic lamina and intimal fibrosis (**463**).

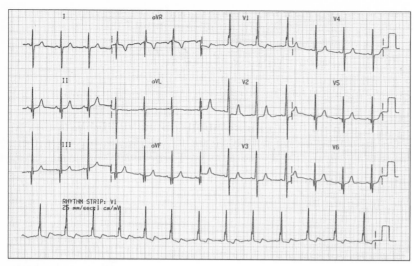

464 Electrocardiogram in primary pulmonary hypertension showing severe right ventricular hypertrophy. There are tall R waves in V1–2 with right axis deviation.

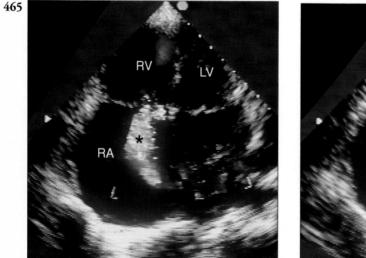

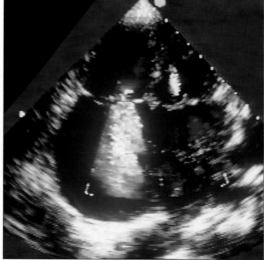

465 & 466 The echocardiogram in heart failure due to pulmonary hypertension may show the cause, but typically there will be dilatation of a hypertrophied right ventricle with tricuspid regurgitation. In this example, both the right atrium and ventricle are enlarged and a jet of regurgitant blood (*)is initially narrow (**465**) and then lengthens and widens later in the cardiac cycle (**466**).

Pulmonary embolism

Pulmonary embolism is one of the commonest causes of acute right heart failure. If the embolism is massive, collapse and shock will ensue. Lesser degrees of pulmonary occlusion may lead to the syndrome of right heart failure. Multiple small emboli may lead to pulmonary hypertension and chronic right heart failure.

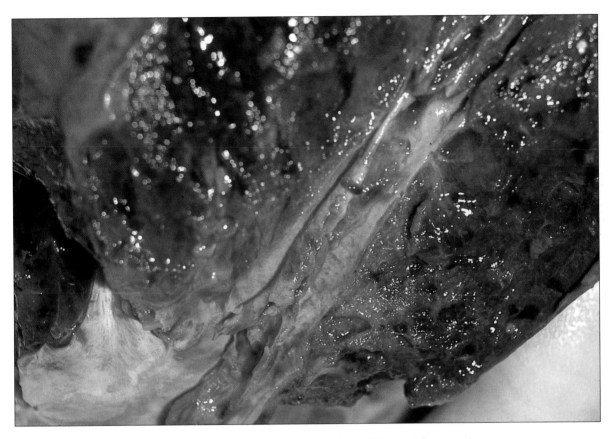

467 Opened lung in a patient who died due to a massive pulmonary embolus filling the left main pulmonary artery.

468 The electrocardiogram in pulmonary embolism may be normal or show a variety of abnormalities. Commonest is said to be the presence of S1, QIII, TIII. This is a response to increased right-sided pressures and raising of the diaphragm. Alternatively, the pattern of acute cor pulmonale may be seen, as in this example, with right atrial enlargement (tall P waves in the inferior leads), right axis deviation and partial right bundle branch block.

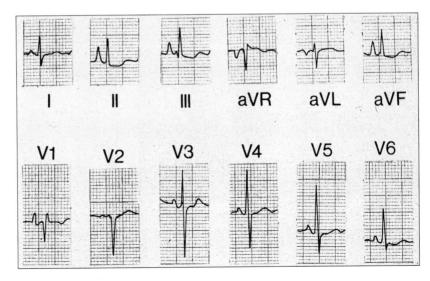

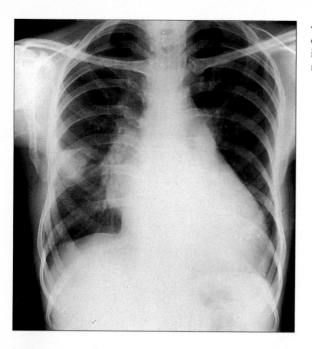

469 There are variety of radiographic appearances in pulmonary embolus, from normal to pulmonary oligaemia. Pulmonary infarction, here seen as a wedge-shaped shadow in the right mid-zone, may herald a massive embolus.

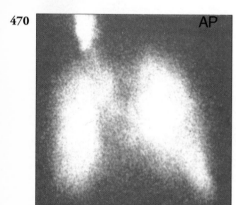

470

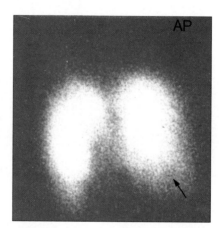

471

470 & 471 Ventilation and perfusion scanning of the lungs is the method of choice for the diagnosis of pulmonary embolus. In this example, in the anterior–posterior projection there is a perfusion defect (arrow, **471**) but normal ventilation at the left lower zone which is virtually diagnostic of embolization.

472

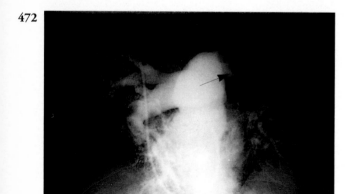

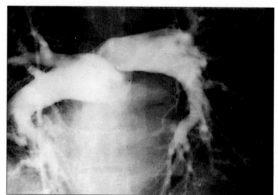

473

472 & 473 Pulmonary angiography showing an embolus filling the right pulmonary artery (arrow) with little distal blood flow (**472**). Following the use of a thrombolytic agent, the obstruction is relieved and blood flow returns to normal (**473**).

REFERENCES

Bonow R. O. *et al.*,1980. Preoperative exercise capacity in symptomatic patients with aortic regurgitation as a predictor of postoperative left ventricular function and long term prognosis. *Circulation*, **62**:1280.

Bonow R. O. *et al.*, 1982. Timing of the operation for aortic regurgitation. *American Journal Cardiology* **50**:325.

Campbell M B., 1970. Natural history of atrial septal defect. *British Heart Journal*, **32**:820.

Codd M. B. *et al.*, 1989. Epidemiology of idiopathic dilated and hypertrophic cardiomyopathy: a population-based studyin Olmstead County, Minnesota 1975-1984. *Circulation*, **80**: 564–572.

Diaz R. A. *et al.* 1987. Prediction of outcome in dilated cardiomyopathy. *British Heart Journal*, **58**:393–9.

Fowler, N. O. 1985. Constrictive pericarditis (physical findings) and Physical findings in cardiac tamponade/The Pericardium in Heart & Disease 1990.

Fuster V. *et al.*,1984. Primary pulmonary hypertension: natural history and the importance of thrombosis. *Circulation*, **70** No 4, 580–587.

Ghali J. K. *et al.*, 1988. Precipitating factors leading to decompensation of heart failure. Archives Internal Medicine, **148**:2013

Ghali J. K. *et al.*, 1990. Trends for hospitalisation rates for heart failure in the USA, 1973–1986. Archives Internal Medicine,**150**:769

Goldman A. P. *et al.*, 1986. Atrial tumours. In *Cancer of the Heart*, ed. Kapoor A. S., Springer–Verlag, New York, p.85

Gradman A. *et al.*, 1989. Predictors of total mortality and sudden death in mid to moderate heart failure. *Journal American College Cardiology*, **14** No. 3, 564–570.

Homans D C, 1985. Current concepts in peripartum cardiomyopathy. *New England Journal Medicine*, **312**:1432

Horstkotte D. *et al.* 1991. Pathomorphological aspects, aetiology and natural history of acquired mitral valve stenosis. *European Heart Journal*,**12** Suppl. B, pp. 55–60.

Kannel W. B. *et al.*, 1988. Cardiac failure and sudden death in the Framingham study. *American Heart Journal* **115**:869

Killip T. *et al.*, 1967. Treatment of myocardial infarction in a coronary care unit. *American Journal Cardiology*, **29**:457.

The Multicenter postinfarction research group (MPRG), 1983. Risk stratification and survival after myocardial infarction. *New England Journal Medicine*, **309**:331–336.

McKee P. A. *et al.*, 1971. The natural history of congestive heart failure: the Framingham study. *New England Journal Medicine* **285**:1441.

McKenna W. J., 1988. The natural history of hypertrophic cardiomyopathy. *Cardiovascular Clin.*, **19**:135.

Newman T. *et al.*, 1988. *Am. J. Med.*, **84 (53A)**: 140.

Roberts W. C. *et al.*, 1977. Sarcoidosis of the heart. *American Journal Cardiology*, **63**:86.

Ross J. & Bramwald E., 1968. The influence of corrective operations on the natural history of aortic stenosis. *Circulation*, **37** (Suppl V) 61.

Rowe J. C. *et al.*, 1960. Course of mitral stenosis without surgery. *Annals of Internal Medicine*, **52**: 741.

Sytkowski P. A. *et al.*, 1990. Changes in risk factors and the decline in mortality from cardiovascular disease. *New England Journal Medicine*, **322**:1635-1641.

Waller B. F. *et al.*, 1982. Aetiology of clinically severe pure mitral regurgitation: analysis of 97 patients over 30 years of age having mitral valve replacement. *American Heart Journal*,**104**:288.

Williams J. B. *et al.*, 1980. Consideration in selection and management of patients undergoing valve replacement with glutaraldehyde–fixed porcine bioprostheses. *Annals Thoracic Surgery*, **30**:247.

Wilson W. R. *et al.*, 1977. Infective endocarditis: a changing spectrum. *Mayo. Clinic. Proceedings*, **52**:254.

Wilson W. R. *et al.*, 1982. Prosthetic valve endocarditis. *Mayo. Clinic. Proceedings*, **57**:155.

Wilson W. R. *et al.*, 1983. Prognosis in severe heart failure: relation to hemodynamic measurements and ventricular ectopic activity. *Journal American College Cardiology*, **2**:403.

INDEX

Numbers in bold print refer to illustrations and their captions.

Abscesses, aortic root 422
Acromegaly 368–371
Alveolitis, fibrosing 354
Amyloidosis 111, 332–339
Anaemia 47
Aneurysms, left ventricular 41, 43,
    101–116
Angiogram
    left ventricular *see* Left ventricular
      angiogram
    pulmonary 472–473
    right ventricular 351
Ankylosing spondylitis 65, 74
    aortic valve 208
Aortic coarctation 150, 451–460
Aortic regurgitation
    acute 79, 227–232
    aortic valve replacement 269–272
    aortography 226, 234–235
    causes 206
    chest radiographs 213–214
    chronic 74, 206–226
    Doppler ultrasound 221–222
    echocardiography 215–220
    haemodynamic tracing 225
    left ventricular cavity dilatation 209
    magnetic resonance imaging 223–224
    pathology 207–209
    phonocardiograms 210–212
    pulses 210–212
Aortic root
    abscess 422
    disease 74, 215–220
Aortic stenosis 65, 179–198
Aortic valve
    ankylosing spondylitis 208
    disease 65, 179–235
    infective endocarditis 409
    prostheses, degeneration 261
    replacement surgery 269–274
    vegetations 419–421
    xenograft infection 425
Aortogram
    aortic regurgitation 226, 234–235
    aortic stenosis 197–198
Atherosclerosis 227
Atrial fibrillation 25, 42, 85
    idiopathic dilated cardiomyopathy
      282
    mitral stenosis 136
    tricuspid stenosis 240
Atrial flutter 32, 41
Atrial septal defect 433–442
Austin Flint murmur 212

Backward failure 11
Balloon valvuloplasty 151–157
Becker's muscular dystrophy 359–360
Bernheim effect 310
Björk–Shiley mitral valve replacement
    268, 330

Bradyarrhythmias 45
Bradycardia 68
Breathlessness (dyspnoea) 13–14
Bundle branch block 65, 67, 340

Cachexia 18
Captopril 7
Carcinoid syndrome 82, 86, 251–254
Cardiac output 1
Cardiac surgery 87, 255–274
Cardiac tamponade 132, 399–407
Cardiomegaly 24, 26, 69, 96
    aortic regurgitation 213–214
    ventricular septal defect 448
Cardiomyopathies 93
    catecholamine 374
    epidemiology 276
    hypertrophic 101, 299–330
    idiopathic dilated 94, 277–294
    idiopathic restricted 113, 340–347
    ischaemic 25
    peripartum 294
    restrictive 111, 332–351
Catecholamine cardiomyopathy 374
Cheilitis 47
Chest radiographs
    acute on chronic renal failure 49–50
    aortic coarctation 456–457
    aortic dissection 229
    aortic regurgitation 213–214
    aortic stenosis 188
    aortic valve replacement 271–272
    atrial septal defect 437
    cardiomegaly 26, 69
    hypertensive heart disease 383
    hypertrophic cardiomyopathy
      314–315
    idiopathic dilated cardiomyopathy
      283–284
    idiopathic restrictive cardiomyopathy
      341
    left ventricular aneurysm 106–107
    mitral regurgitation 166
    mitral stenosis 137
    mitral valvotomy 256–257
    pericarditis 393–394
    pulmonary embolism 469
    sarcoidosis 354
    Starr–Edwards mitral valve replace-
      ment 264–265
    tricuspid stenosis 241
    ventricular septal defect 96, 448
Chordae tendinae, ruptured 49, 58, 174
Clubbing 445
Coarctation of aorta 150, 451–460
Colour flow Doppler
    aortic dissection 232
    aortic root disease 217–220
    aortic stenosis 191
    atrial septal defect 439–440
    hypertrophic cardiomyopathy 317

    mitral regurgitation 169, 171, 173
    subaortic stenosis 203
    supra-aortic stenosis 205
    ventricular septal defect 450
Complete heart block 45, 68
Congenital heart disease 145, 433–460
Continuous wave Doppler
    aortic coarctation 458
    aortic stenosis 193
    hypertrophic cardiomyopathy 321
    idiopathic dilated cardiomyopathy 290
    tricuspid regurgitation 250
Cor pulmonale 468
Coronary arteries
    disease 25–48
    thrombotic occlusion 57–59
Coronary risk factors 53
Computed tomography
    aortic dissection 233
    endomyocardial disease 350
    idiopathic restrictive cardiomyopathy
      344–345
    pericarditis 396
    phaeochromocytoma 373
    pituitary gland 371

Dermal infarcts 412
Doppler ultrasound
    aortic regurgitation 221–222
    mitral stenosis 146–147
    tricuspid stenosis 243
Dyspnoea (breathlessness) 13–14
Dystrophia myotonica 363–364

Early diastolic murmur 184
    subaortic stenosis 199
Ebstein's anomaly 82, 84
Echocardiograms 27–28
    amyloidosis 336–337
    aortic dissection 230–232
    aortic regurgitation 215–220
    aortic stenosis 189–192
    atrial septal defect 438–441
    Björk–Shiley mitral valve replacement
      268
    carcinoid syndrome 254
    endomyocardial disease 349
    Friedreich's ataxia 362
    hypertensive heart disease 384
    hypertrophic cardiomyopathy 316–320
    idiopathic dilated cardiomyopathy
      285–290
    idiopathic restrictive cardiomyopathy
      342–343
    infective endocarditis 415–421
    left atrial myxomata 431–432
    left ventricle 27–28
    left ventricular aneurysm 108–111
    left ventricular function 70–73
    mitral regurgitation 86–87, 167–174
    mitral re-stenosis 258

mitral stenosis 138–145
mitral valve prolapse 259–260
mitral xenograft prolapse 263
myocarditis 298
pericarditis 395
pulmonary hypertension 465–466
rheumatic fever 123–125
right ventricular infarction 119
Starr–Edwards mitral valve replacement 266–267
subaortic stenosis 202–203
supra–aortic stenosis 204–205
tamponade 406–407
tricuspid regurgitation 248–250
tricuspid stenosis 242
valvar infection 425–426
ventricular septal defect 97–99, 449–450
Ehlers–Danlos syndrome 58, 65, 74
Ejection systolic murmur 184
hypertrophic cardiomyopathy 307–308
subaortic stenosis 199
supra–aortic stenosis 200
Electrocardiogram 25
amyloidosis 335
aortic coarctation 454–455
aortic stenosis 186–187
atrial septal defect 436
dystrophia myotonica 364
eosinophilic heart disease 348
hypertensive heart disease 382
hypertrophic cardiomyopathy 311–313
idiopathic dilated cardiomyopathy 282
idiopathic restrictive cardiomyopathy 340
left ventricular aneurysm 104–105
mitral regurgitation 165
mitral stenosis 135–136
myocarditis 297
phaeochromocytoma 374
pulmonary embolism 468
pulmonary hypertension 464
rheumatic fever 122
right ventricular infarction 117–118
supra–aortic stenosis 201
tamponade 404–405
tricuspid stenosis 239–240
ventricular septal defect 447
End-diastolic pressure 1
Endocarditis see Infective endocarditis
Endocrine disorders 368–371
Endomyocardial disease 115, 348–351
Eosinophilic heart disease 348, 351
Epidemiology 8, 4–5
Erythema nodosum 353
Exophthalmos 46

Fabry's disease 365–367
Fatigue 18
Finger clubbing 445
Forward failure 11
Fourth sounds 22, 24, 64, 309, 335
Framingham heart study 3, 56
Friedreich's ataxia 361–362

Gallop rhythm 22
Gated blood pool scanning
left ventricle 29–30
left ventricular aneurysm 113–114
myocardial infarction 76–77
Glycogen storage disorders 365–367

Haemangiomata, perioral 48
Haemochromatosis 365–367
Haemodynamic tracing 31–33
aortic regurgitation 225
aortic stenosis 196
hypertrophic cardiomyopathy 327
mitral regurgitation 91, 176
mitral stenosis 149–150
myocardial infarction 79
tricuspid stenosis 244
Heart failure
causes 24, 51–52
clinical signs 11, 13–24
and coronary risk factors 53
definitions 7, 2
diagnostic criteria 3
epidemiology 8, 4–5
investigations 16, 25–35
precipitating factors 19, 36
prediction of mortality 10–11
presenting features 13
prognosis 6–7, 9
sudden death 8
theoretical progression 12
Heart muscle disease 93, 275
Hepatic congestion 19
Hereditary haemorrhagic telangiectasia 48
Hurler's syndrome 365–367
Hypertension 123, 375–387
pulmonary 153, 461–473
Hyperthyroidism 46
Hypertrophic cardiomyopathy 101, 299–330

Idiopathic dilated cardiomyopathy 94, 277–294
Idiopathic restrictive cardiomyopathy 113, 340–347
Infective endocarditis 137, 408–426
aortic regurgitation 214
tricuspid valve disease 82
Investigations 16, 25–35
Ischaemia 25

Jaundice 19
Jugular venous pressure, elevated 16, 22

Kerley B lines 188
Kussmaul sign 335, 397–398

Left atrial tumours 143, 429–432
Left ventricle
aneurysm 41, 43, 101–116
echocardiogram 27–28
false aneurysm 111
fixed perfusion defect 88–90
hyperdynamic function 323
nuclear imaging 29–30
poor function 25, 53–80

thallium scan 88–90
Left ventricular angiogram 80
hypertrophic cardiomyopathy 328–329
left ventricular aneurysm 115–116
mitral regurgitation 92–93, 177–178
sarcoidosis 355–356
ventricular septal defect 100
Left ventricular failure, acute 39
Left ventricular hypertrophy
amyloidosis 336–337
aortic stenosis 65, 183, 186, 188, 190, 195
Becker's muscular dystrophy 360
hypertensive heart failure 380, 382, 384
hypertrophic cardiomyopathy 301–302, 324–326
idiopathic restrictive cardiomyopathy 344–347
mitral stenosis 135
supra–aortic stenosis 201
Left ventriculography 34–35
idiopathic restrictive cardiomyopathy 346–347
Lungs, ventilation/perfusion scanning 470–471

Magnetic resonance imaging
amyloidosis 338
aortic coarctation 459
aortic regurgitation 223–224
aortic stenosis 195
atrial septal defect 442
hypertensive heart disease 385–386
hypertrophic cardiomyopathy 324–326
idiopathic dilated cardiomyopathy 291–293
ischaemic heart disease 78
left ventricular aneurysm 112
mitral regurgitation 175
mitral stenosis 148
Malar flush 131
Marfan's syndrome 215–220
Mid–diastolic murmur 132–133
Mitral regurgitation 35, 49, 58, 72, 81–93, 125, 158–178
Mitral re–stenosis 255, 257–258
Mitral stenosis 49, 51, 126–157
Mitral valve
Björk–Shiley replacement 268, 330
disease 49, 120–178
floppy 176–178
hypertrophic cardiomyopathy 303
myxomatous change 58
prolapse 58, 259–260
prostheses, degeneration 261–262
Starr–Edwards replacement 264–267
surgery 87, 255–268
vegetations 415–418
xenograft infection 426
xenograft prolapse 263
Mucopolysaccharidosis 365–367
Muscle weakness 18
Muscular dystrophies 359–360

Myocardial infarction 53–80
 anterior 37–39, 65
 anteroseptal 95
 apex cardiogram 64
 arrhythmias 66–67
 cardiac mortality 55
 cardiomegaly 64
 coagulation necrosis 63
 Framingham heart study 56
 inferior 45, 84–85
 Killip classification 54
 left ventricular damage 60–62
Myocardial perfusion scanning (scintigram)
 74–75
Myocarditis 99, 295–298
Myopathy, skeletal 357–358
Myotomy–myectomy 304, 330
Myxomata 143, 427–432

Neuromuscular diseases 118, 357–374

Oedema
 peripheral 17–18
 pitting 17
 pulmonary 383, 457
Orthopnoea 15
Osler's nodes 413

Papillary muscle rupture 81–82
Papilloedema 381
Paroxysmal nocturnal dyspnoea 15
Perfusion defects 74–75
Pericardial effusion 393, 406
Pericarditis 129, 388–398
 cardiac tamponade 401
Peripartum cardiomyopathy 294
Pes cavus 361
Phaeochromocytoma 372–374
Phonocardiograms 20–24
 aortic regurgitation 210–212
 aortic stenosis 184–185
 atrial septal defect 435

mitral regurgitation 83, 162–164
Pituitary gland 371
Pleural effusions 96
 pericarditis 393, 396
 tamponade 406
Pre–systolic murmur 134
Pseudoxanthoma elasticum 58
Pulmonary angiography 472–473
Pulmonary embolism 155, 467–473
Pulmonary hypertension 153, 461–473
Pulmonary oedema 383, 457
Pulmonary plethora 96
Pulmonary wedge pressure, elevated 79,
 91
Pulsed wave Doppler
 aortic stenosis 194
 hypertrophic cardiomyopathy 322
Pulses 20
 aortic coarctation 453
 aortic regurgitation 210–212
Pulsus alternans 21, 33
Pulsus paradoxus
 pericarditis 391–392
 tamponade 402

Reiter's syndrome 65
Renal failure, acute on chronic 49–50
Restrictive cardiomyopathy 111, 332–351
Retina
 aortic coarctation 452
 hypertension 381
Rheumatic fever 49, 84, 120–127
 aortic stenosis 181
Right atrial tumours 143
Right ventricular angiogram 351
Right ventricular hypertrophy
 pulmonary hypertension 465–466
 ventricular septal defect 447
Right ventricular infarction 46, 117–119

Sarcoidosis 117, 352–356
Scintigram 74–75

Sinus rhythm 40
Skeletal myopathy 357–358
Splinter haemorrhages 410–411
Starr–Edwards mitral valve replacement
 264–267
Streptococcus viridans 408
Subaortic stenosis 72, 199, 202–203
Subconjunctival haemorrhage 414
Supra–aortic stenosis 72, 200–201,
 204–205

Tachyarrhythmias 40–44
Tamponade 132, 399–407
Thallium scan 88–90
Third heart sounds 20, 22, 24, 64, 83,
 307
Thromboembolic disease 462–463
Thrombi
 aortic dissection 228
 coronary arteries 57–59
 idiopathic dilated cardiomyopathy
  280, 289, 291–293
 left atrium 144–145
 left ventricular 73, 109
 tamponade 407
Tricuspid valve
 disease 82, 236–254
 regurgitation 82, 84, 23, 245–250
 stenosis 82, 236–244
Tumours 143, 427–432

Valves, prosthetic 255–274
 infection 423–426
Ventilation/perfusion scanning 470–471
Ventricular septal defect 39, 148, 94–100,
 443–450
Ventricular septal hypertrophy 320
Ventricular tachycardia 43–44, 105
Ventriculography 34–35, 346–347